For more healthy lifestyle programs, books, products, and materials by *Jennifer Nicole Lee* please visit:

www.JenniferNicoleLee.com
www.FitnessModelProgram.com
www.BikiniModelProgram.com
www.TheSexyBodyDiet.com
www.JNLCrackTheCode.com
www.GetFitNowWithJNL.com
www.101ThingsNotToDo.com
www.ShopJNL.com
www.MindBodyandSoulDiet.com
www.MindBodyandSoulProgram.com

Praise for *The Mind, Body & Soul Diet*

"If you follow this wonderfully complete program, you will definitely lose weight. I highly recommend it."

—JACK CANFIELD, Co-Author of *The Success Principles* and Co-Founder of the bestselling series *Chicken Soup for the Soul;* featured bestselling Author in *The Secret*

"It's all about working with your mind, body and soul. When you handle all three, you end up with what you've been seeking all along: a fit and fantastic physical being. Jennifer is an expert at teaching just that in this book."

—DR. JOE VITALE, featured bestselling Author in *The Secret*

In The Mind, Body and Soul Diet, *Jennifer Nicole Lee shows us how we can be healthier, healed, and yes happy! Her approach to total well-being is easy to follow, yet yields amazing and powerful results. This is a must read!"*

—MARCI SHIMOFF, #1 NY Times bestselling Author, *Happy for No Reason, Chicken Soup for the Woman's Soul, Chicken Soup for the Mother's Soul,* featured transformational teacher in *The Secret*, www.happyfornoreason.com

"I have learned from Jennifer that health is more than just exercise and eating right - without feeling healthy inside, you have nothing! Jennifer has created a guide for your life to get you and keep you in the right mindset while building a lifestyle around healthy thinking and eating and moving. Let this guide be the plan that brings you to a better self!"

—YOLANDA HARRIS, Former Coaching Sales Manager to Tony Robbins Companies, President, The Keynote Group

"The Mind, Body and Soul Diet *is by far the most empowering and transformational book out there. Jennifer's integrative approach for permanent weight-loss and life fulfillment is comprehensive, inspiring and effective! I would highly recommend this book to my patients and to all those looking to transform their health and their life!"*

—DR. SHAMIRA HUDDA, Founder, Art of Wellness, artofwellness.ca

The
Mind, Body
& Soul Diet

Your Complete Transformational Guide
to Health, Healing, & Happiness

Jennifer Nicole Lee

Cover and back flap photos of JNL by Mike Brochu

Printed in the United States of America.

ISBN: 978-1-48397-092-9

Library of Congress Cataloging-in-Publication Data
Lee, Jennifer Nicole.
The mind, body, & soul diet : your complete transformational guide to health, healing, & happiness / Jennifer Nicole Lee.
    p. cm.
  ISBN 978-1-48397-092-9
  1. Reducing diets. 2. Health. 3. Physical fitness. I. Title.
  RM222.2.L416 2009
  613--dc22
                        2009034598

This publication is designed to provide accurate and authoritative information in regard to the subject matter covered. It is sold with the understanding that the publisher is not engaged in rendering legal, accounting, or other professional services. If legal advice or other expert assistance is required, the services of a competent professional person should be sought.

DEDICATIONS

*This book is dedicated to the person right now reading this:
YOU! May my book bring you health, healing, and happiness
into your life. My book was especially created to help empower,
enlighten, and educate you by being motivated and inspired to
make improvements to increase the quality of your life, forever.*

*I thank my entire book team and management team
who helped me manifest and create this book, which is
to be used as a tool of health, healing, happiness!*

*A sincere thank you to my mom and dad, sisters and
brother, for being an amazing family to me.*

*Thank you to Claudia, Josepha, and Neyda,
for being so loving and caring.*

*Also, thank you to my three kings: my soul mate husband, Edward,
and our two strong and handsome princes, Jaden and Dylan.*

And thank you to my best friend, Marli.

*And thank you to Zan and Mia! The best older brother
and sister that Jaden and Dylan could ever have.*

*I would like to also thank the pioneers and teachers of light who
have passed on before me and who are still living now, helping me
to enjoy the success which I have created to be where I am today.*

ACKNOWLEDGMENTS

Creating a book is one of the most magical experiences, one which requires a collective effort by many, with many goals in mind; to empower, enlighten, educate, and entertain the reader. I could not have created this book without the help of my many editors and my publisher who believed in its message and mission to help others. I would also like to acknowledge my business partners, Fitness Brands, Inc. and Tara Productions who helped to spread the word to the world of our impressive record of fitness successes. And of course, I thank my staff at JNL, Inc. who day in and day out share in the miracles we help create in so many of our clients lives.

In particular, I would like to thank my Higher Power for guiding me daily to make the right decisions in life and to lead me on the right path. My entire heart pours out to family with love: my soul mate, Edward, for his unfailing love and support, and my sons, Jaden and Dylan, for giving me the joy of motherhood with their laughter and light, and for teaching me the real meaning and purpose of life. My family is my rock and my greatest success. And I could not have achieved what I have, without the dedication of my best friend and executive assistant, Marli.

I would also like to thank all of my associates in the fitness/wellness, self-help, and life coaching industries, who contributed their expertise to make this book complete and comprehensive, as well as those self-help/metaphysical authors and teachers who have paved the way for me, and the many other "crusaders of light."

I would like to thank Tara, for her angelic attitude, sweet spirit, miracle-believing outlook on life, and loving generosity. To baby Skye

Madison, for being such a blessing to all of our lives. To Elisa, for being a truly devoted professional who is so fun to work with. To Michael, a seasoned expert with whom I've had the opportunity to work on globally successful fitness products. To David, for believing in me on both a personal and professional level, and being so wonderful to work with. These wonderful people are angels for believing in me, and allowing me to share my passion for fitness and living a healthy lifestyle with the world.

A big "thank you" to my personal trainer and coach, William Del Sol, who pushes me up and out of my comfort zone every time we train— and who never allows me to fail myself. Lastly, I would like to thank all of my past, present, and future fitness friends, for allowing me to motivate, empower, and enlighten them. I believe in you!

TABLE OF CONTENTS

FOREWORD

by Bestselling Author,
Dr. Joe Vitale of *The Secret*

When Jennifer asked me to write the foreword to this book, I almost said no. I'm too busy with travels and books of my own. But I've seen her on television, glanced at her websites, and knew this was a woman with passion and wisdom. So I said I'd take a look at her book. I'm glad I did.

This book is packed with insights, tips, ideas and methods to help you do one thing: get healthy. But please note that this is not a one-sided approach to "healthy." This isn't just about looking good in a bathing suit. This is about feeling good about your body, your life and yourself. This is a well-rounded, inside-out approach to transforming your entire life.

If you want proof that the wisdom in this incredible book works, just look at Jennifer. Her work is in over 100 different countries world-wide (from Europe, to Asia, South America, etc). And you may have seen the infomercial marketing her as a Fitness Celebrity Expert and a weight loss success story. She's gorgeous, successful, productive, prolific and — above all — happy.

And that's the key; you want to take care of your inner life — your well-being — while you take care of your outer life — your body. It's all about working with your mind, body and soul. When you handle all three, you end up with what you've been seeking all along: a fit and fantastic physical being. Jennifer is an expert at teaching just that.

I love Jennifer's book. It's her voice and wisdom in a simple, easy, direct form. You'll feel as if she is sitting beside you, talking right to you, as you read her book. You can read this book quickly, but I urge you not to. Instead, savor this material. Read with a pen in hand. Underline passages. Take notes. And act on what you learn.

I was in the movie *The Secret*, which was about transforming your life by learning the Law of Attraction. Well, if *The Secret* was about weight loss, it would be this book. Jennifer's wonderful book is going to stand out years from now as a classic in health and fitness literature. But the book is far more than a guide to getting trim. It's actually a guide to transforming your life. I love it, and know you will, too.

Read and be well.

Happy Transforming!
Dr. Joe Vitale
www.mrfire.com

See Your Doctor First

The information and advice given in this book are not intended as substitutes for medical advice or diagnosis. It is designed solely to provide helpful information on the subjects addressed. This book is sold with the understanding that the author and publisher are not rendering medical, health, or other personal services. Please consult with your physician before starting the Mind, Body and Soul Diet, and also before changing your diet or exercise routine. You should rely on your physician's advice regarding whether the Mind, Body and Soul Diet is appropriate for you and you should rely on your physician to establish your weight goal. The author, persons mentioned in this book, and publisher disclaim all liability associated with the recommendations and guidelines set forth in this book.

Pre-Mind, Body & Soul Diet Consultation

One of the most important aspects to address before starting a complete transformational health program is preparing yourself for the miracles that are going to come your way. As a life coach, I spend an immense amount of time with my personal clients, getting them ready for the amazing journey ahead of them. I have found, through my experience, that the key to achieving magical results is to make sure my clients are mentally prepared and committed to making these improvements in their lives.

You see, merely being interested in a thing is a wholly different mindset than being committed to it. In order for you to create positive transformations, you must be committed to making the necessary changes in your life that will yield successes. How do I get you prepared? By making sure you are fully focused, dedicated, and ready to take on your brand-new life.

How do you get to this point? I like to take my personal clients through an exercise I call the "Pre-Mind, Body and Soul Consultation." In this exercise, take some quiet time to carefully consider your past and present states. Ask yourself these empowering questions:

1. If I continue with my current lifestyle, where will I be in one year? Two years? Five years? And 10 years?

2. Is what I am doing currently working for me, or against me?

3. Am I living my life to its utmost potential?

4. If I don't make the necessary changes in my life, starting today, where will my life end up?

5. Am I totally, fully happy with my life now?

6. Am I ready to prove to myself, my family, and the world just how amazing I am?

7. Do I accept that, in order to become an example of personal excellence, I must go above and beyond my own expectations, and also the expectations of others?

8. Up until now, have I really amazed myself and those close to me with my own abilities?

9. Do I understand that, to be a winner, I must learn from other winners?

10. Do I fully comprehend that during my journey to become my best, there will be times of frustration and growing pains, through which I must perservere in order to achieve my desired results?

While following the Mind, Body and Soul Diet program, you'll experience a new level of excitement thanks to your changed lifestyle and fitness freedom. You will be blessed with the energy that comes from health, healing and happiness. But you may also experience down times, difficulties and challenges. Be steadfast! Stay focused on your goals. Remember, keeping your eye on the prize is essential to your victory. Many will try to distract you and deter you. Visit back to your Mind, Body and Soul Diet principles—and rededicate yourself to your goals.

At times, you may feel that you are moving too slowly towards your desired outcomes. You may ask yourself "Why haven't I lost weight yet? Why isn't this working faster? Why don't I have the body of my dreams by now?" When these negative feelings boil up, remind yourself that success doesn't happen overnight. Striving for personal excellence in all areas of your life takes patience and persistence. If you have to undo years of inward and outward resistance and negative conditioning, it will take more time.

Just sit back, relax, take a big, deep breath in and then exhale. You are about to embark on one of the most magical and miraculous times of your life. Just know that you will reach your goals, if you stick to the principles outlined in this book. Like my own transformation, it won't happen overnight—but it will happen! Because I refused to give up or give in, I've been given the gift to motivate you to create your dream life. I'm proud to pass the torch of wisdom to you, so that you too can succeed in all areas of your life—through health, healing and happiness.

If you're getting results, but you hit a plateau, don't let it sap your motivation. It's only natural to hit plateaus. Think of it as a "rest area" to ramp up for the amazing benefits to come. It's like pulling into a rest stop on a long road trip, a pause to refuel and get re-organized for the remainder of your journey. Don't waste your time getting frustrated. Plateaus happen to everyone, in every aspect of life—especially when you are learning something new. Success comes in waves, like the ocean. So, when a wave of success is on its way out, use that down time to strategize and prepare for your continued progress.

As anyone who has ever learned to play a new sport, or a musical instrument, or gone to college to learn a new trade, will tell you, there is always a learning curve, and plateaus along the way. It's how you handle this experience that separates the losers from the winners. A winner is the loser who picks herself up that one last time, and continues on. So keep plugging through. This is when you must be committed to your success, not just interested.

"The best way to live the life of your dreams is to start living the life of your dreams TODAY, in every little way that you possibly can." —MIKE DOOLEY, featured bestselling author in *The Secret*

PREFACE & WELCOME TO THE MIND, BODY & SOUL DIET

I warmly welcome you to my innovative, productive, and complete lifestyle program: *The Mind, Body & Soul Diet; Your Complete Transformational Guide to Health, Healing & Happiness.* If you have been seeking to create a healthy balance in your life, but have found that hard to accomplish in an unbalanced world, you have the right book in your hands.

Yes, this book contains a "diet." In fact, it's a complete lifestyle guide to follow for increased health and vitality. But don't get me wrong, it's not a traditional "diet." I actually dislike diets, and dieting—and you probably do, too. After all, what are the first three letters of the word "diet"? D-I-E. Exactly. *Die*! And we don't want to die. We want to live – and eat, and exercise for optimal health. I have been on too many different diets which caused me to yo-yo up and down on the scale, losing weight only to gain it all back, and then some. The only program that has allowed me, and many others who have also experienced diet relapse, to lose weight and keep it off, is the Mind, Body and Soul Diet. With it, you will finally crack your weight loss code and keep the weight off forever, while enjoying the process.

What makes this diet so much more evolved and effective than others is my approach to complete wellness and wholeness of the mind, body and soul. And I chose the word *diet* because I *do* want you to be on a diet; not just rejecting bad food choices, but also unhealthy, self-sabotaging behaviors. I want you to be on a diet from non-productive habits, like failing to prepare and eating "accidentally." With this book, you will be shown how to be on a diet that frees you from outdated belief systems, harmful thoughts, and parasitic people who don't help but hinder you. I'm here to get you off of an unhealthy diet, and onto a healthy one. Remember that diet you went on, that cut out sugar and carbs? Well, *The Mind, Body & Soul Diet* will teach you to cut out unhealthy practices, false principles, and archaic habits that work against you, not for you.

This diet is revolutionizing the weight loss industry with its three-pronged approach to health, healing and happiness. Everyone, from multi-tasking modern moms, to doctors and leading fitness experts, is falling back in love with being fit, because the Mind, Body and Soul Diet works! Let me show you why.

Your Mind: Why address the mind? Because your mind is the control center of your reality. Your mind controls your focus, your emotions, and your attention. Your mind is the strongest "muscle" in your body; the more you use it, the stronger it gets. It creates positive thoughts, or forces you to dwell in negativity, destroying joy. Putting your mind on a diet free of negative thoughts, negative images, and negative self-talk is a must, if you want to experience true health, healing and happiness.

Your Body: Why address the body? Because your body is a holy shrine, a glorious creation which no unclean thing should sully. It needs to be treated with love and respect in order to be healthy, healed, and happy.

Your Soul: Why address the soul? Because spiritual well-being is an integral part of mental, emotional, and physical health. Spirituality and faith provide you with the means with which to detach yourself from your current stifling and stressful circumstances, and give you the clarity with which to observe your life as a true miracle. Your life will be richer, you will be more balanced, and experience inner peace, when you nurture your spirit and feed your soul, thus being healthy, healed, and happy.

Your Health: Why address health? I know you have heard the saying "If you don't have your health, you don't have anything." Nothing could be more true. Think back to the last time you were really ill. When you are sick, it feels like the end of the world. You're depressed, weak, and drained. It's plain that your health should be your most prized possession. Treat it with respect, and you'll experience a quantum leap in vitality. When we are healthy, we feel unstoppable.

Your Healing: Why address healing? Because the spiritual act of healing yourself is essential to self-growth and personal improvement. Being healed liberates you. Healing yourself gives you priceless personal freedom; freedom from hurtful events in the past and bad memories. We may not realize it, but we allow past negative events to replay over and over in our present lives, hindering us from progressing. When you practice daily rituals of self-healing, you become whole and balanced. And when you are whole and balanced, you have control of your life and, more importantly, of your emotions. Not allowing your emotions to control you will also stop emotional eating, which is one of the main contributors to becoming overweight. Once you are healed, and work daily at healing yourself, you will not eat emotionally, and will enjoy lifelong weight loss and health.

Your Happiness: Why address happiness? Because isn't being happy what life is all about? Having pure, real, authentic joy in our lives is our natural birthright. One of the things we're apt to forget along the path of life is that it's not about the destination, but the journey. This is the secret to the Mind, Body and Soul Diet. Being healthy is not a one-time event, but a journey to be enjoyed along the way, one day at a time.

The key to lifelong weight loss is mastering the Mind, Body and Soul Diet

We all have lost weight before, only to gain it back. It's called "diet relapse." We gain the weight back because we've taken a temporary, band aid approach to a complex problem. *The Mind, Body & Soul Diet* delves deeper. With it, you will not only lose weight, but learn how to master lifelong weight control, achieve personal healing, and celebrate life with days of happiness.

"Slow and steady wins the race"

—A E S O P, *teacher of moral lessons, taken from the fable of "The Tortoise and the Hare" 620-560BC*

As a wellness guru, I see living a healthy lifestyle not as just something you do, then are done with. Rather, being healthy is a lifelong goal, reached one day at a time. You will come to savor this journey of creating your optimal health, because you have seen for yourself that the quick and easy route doesn't take you where you want to go. Not only does it not last, the quick-fix actually backfires, slowing down your metabolism and, ultimately, negatively impacting your confidence level and spirit. Slow and steady is the way to lasting results, and I'll guide you every step of the way.

First of all, I don't want you to rush into weight loss. Quick weight loss is not healthy, and will not serve you in the long run. I'll show you many ways to increase your vitality through invigorating exercises, and delicious life-boosting foods chock full of anti-aging and disease-fighting antioxidants. You will be taught self-mastery, as you learn how to heal yourself from emotional stress, painful past events, and bad memories that have scarred your spirit. Our wounded souls are stained by old traumas which have left us in physical, emotional, and psychological distress. But we have the power within ourselves to heal our souls, and to move on and up.

As you can see, this is not just your typical next, new, hot fad diet. It's not filled with the shallow lies that we've all been told, like "eat this and do that, and you will lose weight." If you have lost weight only to gain it all back with the one-dimensional approach of calorie-in/calorie-out, now you will be shown a better way. Even if this is your first time trying to lose weight, this is still the right book for you. You will learn how to build health on a solid foundation, learning lifelong health principles and anti-aging rituals that won't ever fail you.

My *Mind, Body and Soul Diet* is revolutionizing the health industry, and will change the way people approach losing weight forever, because no other program combines and addresses the importance of all three components of health. In this diet, it's all covered: the physical aspects of exercising, eating optimally, and the importance of learning to have self-governance over our emotions. No other "diet" has shown us how to use the power of our minds to enjoy lifelong health benefits like this, to increase the quality of our lives, long term. Last but not least, this book also covers the much-overlooked, yet so important, spiritual component to complete wellness. I am here to say, loud and proud, that losing weight, getting in shape and being your best YOU is a spiritual journey. By including the spiritual aspect in achieving permanent weight loss you will learn how to nurture your soul and reawaken your dormant passions, making your life much richer and more meaningful. You will reconnect with your Higher Power, and become more spiritual and connected to the Universe, by being inspired to practice simple yet powerful daily activities such as meditating and living in a constant state of gratitude. You will experience an increase in your energy, endurance, and stamina. You will discover a new-found sense of mental, emotional, physical, and spiritual freedom in your life.

"You are only as old as you feel." —ANONYMOUS

The benefits of this diet are bountiful; turning back the clock of age with a toned, athletic body, flexible joints, a sound mind, and razor-sharp focus, plus a glowing complexion that radiates optimal health. You'll discover healing tools and timeless principles that you can use to nurture your own health, restore your balance, and create greater joy and fulfillment in your life.

Over the years I have done many weight loss, fitness, and life coaching consultations with people of differing backgrounds, from all around the world. My clients have not only successfully lost weight, but have started practicing priceless success principles in their lives, and have been able to learn true self-mastery, the mastery over emotions and the mind, thus liberating them of self-inflicted emotional warfare, hurtful thoughts, and negative self-talk.

I have seen miracles happen through the Mind, Body and Soul Diet. Actually, I am my own first miracle. I yo-yoed up and down in my weight and on the scale most of my life. Unstable in my emotions, with a negative mindset, no confidence and low self-esteem, I allowed these factors to govern my life and my actions. Through my Mind, Body and Soul Diet, I was finally able to take hold of my life, from controlling my weight, to controlling my mind and emotions. So, take comfort and be confident that the Mind, Body and Soul Diet will work for you, too, because I am not speaking only about principles, but from my personal experience, when I tell you that it works. The Mind, Body and Soul Diet principles have worked for me and my many clients from around the world, and they will work for you too!

The principles always worked—but you have to work the principles.

"A key can unlock a door.
But you have to pick up the key to use it."
—JENNIFER NICOLE LEE

All of your life's dreams, weight loss, and health goals are possible. I know for a fact, beyond a shadow of a doubt, that you too can achieve your healthy heart's desire, with the Mind, Body and Soul Diet principles. But here is the key: the principles work, but you have to work the principles. Please visit www.MindBodyandSoulProgram.com to listen to real-life testimonials from women who have used these principles, and who have made life-changing improvements in their lives.

A year ago, I was on a television show. I had made the bold, confident, yet true claim that anyone who applied the universal principals, found in the book which you are holding, would experience lifelong weight loss, achieve balance in their life in an unbalanced world, find inner peace in an unpeaceful world. They would never again suffer from uncontrollable emotional eating, would get in amazing shape, and would enjoy the entire journey. The interviewer was very critical and skeptical of my message. After the interview, she confided in me that she had just gone through a horrendous divorce and was suffering from depression and anxiety. She had gained over 35 pounds in less than 6 months, had lost her zest in life, and her job was on the line after receiving 2 warnings. I told her that I would coach her privately, but she had to use the principals. After I worked with her for only 3 private sessions, she went on to make some very big miracles happen in her life. And the best part is that it only took only seven short months to manifest them all. Yes, all of these great miracles didn't happen in 2 weeks, but they did happen. Today she is in the best shape of her life. She lost 40 pounds, gained a whole new perspective, is in a loving, supportive, joyful relationship, and ended up moving on to a bigger and better position at a new job, making a much better salary. I recently caught up with her, and guess what? The miracles are still happening in her life, as the Mind, Body and Soul Diet principles you will find in this book are still working for her, and she is now on her upward spiral of success.

So what makes my Mind, Body and Soul Diet so powerful? It's that my technique to permanent and lifelong weight loss and health relies upon addressing three main aspects of your being, creating complete balance:

- **The Mind:** by positively directing it to control your emotional states and thus utilizing true self-mastery; learning how to make your mind your best friend, supportive and full of self-love and self-respect—rather than your own worst enemy, critical and negative.

- **The Body:** by treating and respecting it like a sacred holy entity, a housing place for the mind and soul. You will give your body gifts of exceptional nutrition and exhilarating exercises which will bless it, detox it, and cleanse it from the inside out.

- **The Soul:** you will enjoy engaging in soul-awakening practices which will motivate and inspire you to a higher spiritual level, giving you strength and support to continue your journey.

My *Mind, Body* & Soul Diet will increase your quality of life in so many ways:

- Finally you will be able to find balance in an unbalanced world, peace in an unpeaceful world, quiet in your mind which previously experienced inner mental civil war, and clarity in a once-cluttered spiritual state.

- You will, once and for all, gain control over your emotions, stopping and banishing all emotional eating.

- You will finally start eating healthier, exercising more and, surprisingly, enjoying your newfound fitness freedom.

- You will connect with your Higher Power, awaken your helpful and powerful alter ego, and rediscover your true passions in life.

- You will be excited to wake up in the morning thanks to the new goals you've set into motion, your new exercise program, and your revved-up metabolism.

- You will gain the tools that you need to create and master lifelong weight-loss success.

- You will live life with boundless energy, feeling younger and full of ageless energy!

- Anti-aging beauty rituals will become a part of your everyday new healthy habits, and you will "grow younger," diminishing the visible signs of aging and stress.

- You will feed your spirit daily, to continue on your life and fitness journey.

- You will be constantly inspired and empowered from within to be your very best.

So, wipe away all the useless diet advice you have been told before, and embrace this book. Enjoy learning how to celebrate being fit and healthy, one day at a time with universal fitness truths. My book is one of the greatest gifts you could give yourself, or give to anyone that you love or want to help. The more you read it, the more priceless information you will find, and the fitter, healthier, and younger you will become! The more you refer back to this diet, the more you'll understand that it's fun to be fit! The more you read, the more you'll celebrate fitness in your life instead of viewing it as a burden.

Realize that you're giving yourself the greatest present of all; the gifts of a healthy lifestyle, exercise, nutrient-rich foods, and anti-aging rituals full of healing benefits. Realize that fitness starts in the mind, and then flows throughout the body. Congratulations to your new healthy, healed, happy, and younger YOU! Cheers to your health!

CHAPTER 1

Wellness Is a Journey to be Enjoyed

"You have one life to live, but if you live it right, to your fullest, healthiest potential, then once is enough." —JENNIFER NICOLE LEE

Everyone is the author of her own book of their life. Sadly, the chapters most commonly written are work, stress, strife, depression, lack, and drama. I'm an Ambassador of Balance and Wellness, urging all to write lengthy chapters of health, prosperity, joy, self-love, and self respect, to achieve complete balance of wellness." —JENNIFER NICOLE LEE

J ust as this book has many chapters, so does your life. You will read this book one word at a time, one page at a time; and so you must also take life one page at a time. So right now, take a big, deep breath in and exhale slowly. Relax a bit, and understand that being healthy is not a wind-sprint or a marathon, but a well-paced "jog" to be celebrated at every milestone and landmark.

We members of the human race suffer from what I call "I-want-it-now-itis" and "get-there-now-itis." By that, I mean that we're stuck in the here and now. This "I-have-to-have-it-now" mentality will not serve you or move you forward. It will only frustrate you and lead you to lose your energy and focus. When we cage ourselves into that kind of limited thinking, it's impossible to enjoy the journey of life one day at a time, one goal at a time. In America especially we live at a super-fast pace. This is why our premature mortality rate is so high, and our health is so poor. From my extensive research and travels to areas in the world such as Asia and Europe, I witnessed firsthand how obesity is rare and longevity is common. The pace of life there is much more relaxed and balanced, the food is not as processed, and exercise is a part of everyday life.

As a Certified Life Coach, I see this "race to the finish-line" mentality all the time in counseling sessions. It affects people from all walks of life. It even once affected me. Even though I'm an author, a lifestyle consultant, and a weight-loss success story myself, I too suffered from this hindering and unhelpful mindset. But before I was able to achieve many life goals, I had to force myself out of my own comfort zone and move from an "I want it now" mentality to one that recognizes life as an enjoyable journey to be traveled one day at a time with a long-term goal in mind.

You should think of fitness and anti-aging rituals as constant daily practices, not just something you do once. For example, we can't go to the gym once and then become instantly healthy. We can't meditate once and then be balanced and enlightened spiritually for the rest of our lives. Rather, if we take the long view regarding our health, healing, and happiness, and finding true joy one day at a time, one moment at a time, we can turn our unsuccessful life into an extremely successful and fulfilling one, filled with health, wholeness, and happiness.

Our life and our health are the greatest gifts we've been given. Being healthy cannot be achieved in a one-time effort. A healthy, whole and happy life is achieved by many steps, taken one at a time. It's up to you to point yourself toward the destination of your choice. Life should not to be rushed, but is meant to be celebrated, relished, and embraced.

A New Outlook = A New Look

In order for me to enjoy a healthy lifestyle and make the right conscious decisions every day, I had to make some fundamental changes in my outlook. Before I did, I was miserable. I didn't feel good. My outlook on life was bleak. I didn't have the energy or passion for life that I do now, and I remember how down and bad I felt. I know first-hand how living an unhealthy lifestyle brought me certain consequences, like lack of stamina, no endurance, and no real joy for life. But since I made the decision to implement my own *Mind, Body and Soul Diet* principles in my life, I have enjoyed tremendous benefits, such as sleeping better, feeling fit, having more endurance to keep up with the demands of my busy life, and also looking younger. I'm in my — uh, should I say mid-thirties? — and I actually feel younger with more energy and passion then I did in my early twenties. It's hard to believe that, just a short few years ago, I felt as if I was in my sixties! I wore a plus-size wardrobe, and I didn't even have children yet. I had no excuses, but I played the victim. I felt trapped by the limitations of my weak, unhealthy mind and quickly aging body. I was mystified by all the contradictory weight loss information out there. So I feel your pain and I know your confusion.

Conditioned, Programmed, and Raised to Be Fat

I grew up in a first-generation Italian family, and the first question my mother asked my brother, sisters, and me every morning was, "So what would you like to eat today?" From birth, I was bombarded with the conception that eating a lot of food is very important, and was the focus of our day.

There was no doubt that, as I child, I was loved through food. I learned from my parents that food was the beginning and the end, the alpha and the omega. We seemed to eat all the time. We ate when we were happy, sad, bored, tired, or stressed, and we ate when we weren't even hungry. This came from the old paradigm of how my parents were raised, that eating equaled survival. And forget eating for health! According to this type of archaic mentality, as long as there was food on the table, and lots of it, you were "successful" and going to survive.

Even though being raised in a beautiful, rural Southern town was a great experience in many ways, I was also something of an outcast. I was dark, with olive-toned skin, and we were the only ones with the very Italian last name, Siciliano. Funny to think about it, but my family and I kind of stuck out. I never really felt like I belonged or fit in.

So, who were my friends? Who could I rely upon? A hot, steaming plate of spaghetti and meatballs, which always seemed to be ready in our home. Needless to say, I coped by doing a lot of emotional eating. My weight yo-yoed up and down a lot because the only way I knew how to lose weight was to go on the latest fad diet. I tried the "orange and toast diet," "cabbage soup diet," and every other low-calorie diet everyone else was trying. This cycle was lonely and desperate, being wrapped in that instant, emotional comfy blanket of macaroni and cheese or homemade pizza, then subjecting myself to self-enforced scarcity just to lose weight.

It wasn't until tragedy impacted my life that I stopped spiraling downwards and started spiraling *upwards*. I had met the most wonderful man ever, my husband, when I was on the heavier side of the scale, about 170 pounds. We fell in love, got married, and then we decided to start a family. But our rosy start to marriage was interrupted by tragedy; I miscarried during my first pregnancy. Not only did I lose the life of my unborn baby, I almost lost my own life because I was in very bad physical shape. I knew at that moment—that proverbial "ah-ha" moment—that not only did I have to get healthy for myself once and for all, but I had to get healthy for my future family so I could be the fittest mother to my kids and the best wife ever to my husband.

That's what led me to begin the journey towards improving my lifestyle. It's not really about looking good in a bikini; it's not about a number on a scale or a certain dress size. It's not even about losing weight, because when you lose something, you subconsciously go looking for it. I've lost weight in the past so many times, only to find it back on my body.

It's not about loss; if you want to get healthy, it's about gaining. I have lost weight, but I've gained so much more. I've gained a new identity as an athlete. I've gained the energy to run around with my kids. I've gained the mental fortitude to never give up or give in. I've gained the super-productive mindset that it's not about perfection, but rather about persistence. I've gained the stamina to take on life and do what I want to do. I've gained the endurance to achieve my life's goals. I've gained the "I-can-do-it" attitude, the mental fortitude, and the emotional strength that I need, to not only reach my weight loss goals but also my life goals. With the *Mind, Body, and Soul Diet*, you can, too. This book is not about trimming down a bit, but about a complete transformation dedicated to your health, healing, and happiness.

Transformational Health

"Your body is not a mechanical structure fixed in time and space. It is a field of energy, information, and intelligence in dynamic exchange with your environment, capable of perpetual healing, renewal, and transformation."
—DEEPAK CHOPRAH, M.D., *Foremost*
Pioneer in Integrated Medicine

Transformational health integrates the wellness practices of the mind, the body, and the soul, thus creating a complete, balanced and whole life, full of radiating health. Transformational health is much more in-depth than the simplistic thinking of calorie-in/calorie-out. We have been misled by society, doctors, and other so-called fitness gurus to think if we just eat this food and do this exercise, we'll be healthy. Real transformational health is so much more than that.

Complete transformational health involves:

- healing yourself from past negative events so you can move forward
- getting control over the strongest muscle of your body, your mind
- making your emotions work for you, not against you
- discovering spiritual well-being and understanding that you are never alone in your journey in life

- permanently adding mind-boosting foods and supplements into your diet to help prevent mental illness, depression, and anxiety

- enjoying daily beauty rituals to help you look and feel your best

- eating foods and performing exercises that actually reverse the signs of aging, and boost your energy levels, helping you to feel your youngest, most vibrant best

Transformational health is more metaphysical than just staying away from sugar, or eating a low-carb diet. It starts in the mind and flows throughout your body. That means that whatever happens in your mind, will manifest in your body. If you think unhealthy, negative thoughts, you will become unhealthy and negative, bitter and sour, and just plain miserable.

But, if you start cleaning your "mental house" by gaining clarity about what you want, and letting go of archaic behaviors, belief systems, thoughts, ideas, and people that don't help you but hinder you, you will experience a complete transformation in your life.

"Our deepest fear is not that we are inadequate. Our deepest fear is that we are powerful beyond measure. It's our light, not our darkness, that most frightens us. We ask ourselves, who am I to be brilliant, gorgeous, talented, and fabulous? Actually, who are you not to be? You are a child of God. Your playing small doesn't serve the world. There's nothing enlightened about shrinking so that other people won't feel insecure around you. We are all meant to shine, as children do. And as we let our own light shine, we unconsciously give other people permission to do the same." —MARIANNE WILLIAMSON

This is difficult for people to understand and embrace because they are afraid of their own brilliance. We all fail in our lives; it is how we learn. However, it's not failure that we're most afraid of. Rather, we are most fearful of our own true abilities, our own brilliance, and our own light. We've sadly seen many times in our lives that if we let our light shine, other people may not like us. After all, the saying goes "misery loves company." But I want to encourage, support and help you to finally break from the miserable pack and discover your true identity as the new super-healthy and prosperous you.

"Your current state doesn't have to be your fate."
—JENNIFER NICOLE LEE

The state that you're in right now does not have to be your destiny. As I like to say, your current state is not your fate. It's only temporary. For example, look at a caterpillar. It goes through some very interesting stages and challenges, before it becomes a beautiful butterfly. So you, too, will go through changes, stages which you must pass through, before morphing into your best you.

We all get fed up and frustrated when we seem to be stuck in the here and now. We sometimes feel as if we are going nowhere fast. But we must understand that our current situation is not our future. We must broaden our vision, and see what lies beyond the horizons if we want to become successful, happy and fit.

This is not a "do-over"diet, as in, if you do it again, it will help you lose weight again. We have all done too many "do-over" diets. Rather, the Mind, Body and Soul Diet, is a complete "make-over" diet, where you will fall back in love with being you and being fit, living life with lifelong benefits.

As a life coach, I am here to remind you that you do indeed have the power to create the rest of your life exactly how you want it. We often forget our own power. I am here to wake you up, to take you out of your own busy routine, to take your head out of the sand, and unplug you from complacency. I am going to steer you to success and a better life. But you must fight for your right to get fit, and stay there. And now is the best time to break your own addiction to mediocrity, to fitting in with those who are miserable around you.

"You are not born with confidence.
You must create it from within." —J N L

"Faith is essential. When no one else believes in
you, you must have faith in your own abilities,
and lean on your Higher Power." —J N L

By reading this book, you are reconnecting with the real, true, wonderful inner you that is just so eager to come out. This is the tipping point for you. To counteract all your negative messages, from now on, I want you to take your Vitamin C—and I'm not talking about the Vitamin C you get from orange juice or a multivitamin—I'm talking vitamin C for Confidence. And you know what else? I want you to use the F-word more than ever—and I'm not talking profanity—I'm talking about Faith.

Here is my equation for results:

Vitamin C (CONFIDENCE) + the F-Word (FAITH) = RESULTS

Vitamin C plus the F-word equals results. Take your confidence and use your faith every day, and you'll get results. But how do we get confidence, and enough faith to make miracles happen in our lives? Well, we don't just sit around wishing and hoping for it. We must create it in our own physiology.

"Pretend until you are not pretending anymore." —J N L

"The body doesn't lie."—J N L

How do we build up our own inner confidence and faith? The same way we build up our muscles—by exercising them! So here is an exercise for you. Start with your "Superman Walk." Think of an imaginary cape flowing off your back in the wind. Your have great posture with your abs in and your head held high. Your shoulders are back, your chest is out proudly, and your chin is up. When you walk, walk with a definite purpose. This is a power-stance that will start you on your upward spiral. When you walk, tell yourself that you are worthy of a new, better, healthier, whole, fulfilling, prosperous, joyful life-style filled with endless abundance and health—and allow your body to illustrate these powerful messages. You deserve it! Use this power exercise daily—it really works. Sometimes we tell ourselves that we are confident, but we don't feel it. By controlling our physiology, our body, and putting it into a powerful position with this Superman Walk, we do feel more confident, instantly!

Molly, one of my most challenging clients, had one of the most horrific life stories that I had ever heard. Without going into detail, I can tell you that I was frankly shocked that she was still alive and functioning after all that she had gone through. Nonetheless, with my Mind, Body and Soul Diet principles, and my constant life coaching, she was able to blast through the limitations that life had placed on her. She now is a living example of what confidence, faith, and a support group can help you to achieve.

I believed in Molly, even though she didn't believe in herself. So I urge you reading this book, to have faith in yourself. Having faith means to believe in things which can't be seen, but which you know are true. So believe in yourself, that you can and will achieve your new healthy lifestyle. You have the tools, tips and techniques right here to manifest the results that you desire and deserve in your life. That you are reading this book right now is proof that you do have faith. You are headed in the right direction. And I have faith in you, too. I, as your life coach, am holding you accountable. Use the timeless, tried and true principles in this book to help you positively progress.

"A gift comes in every mistake and failure.
It's the gift of learning a lesson, of what not to
do next time, and how to do it better." —JNL

This book is my gift to you. You will be shown what, and what not, to do. Most of you have made the same mistakes that I have, so you are not alone. And many of you are just beginning, so you don't have to make all my mistakes that I did. That's the beauty of the fitness friendship that I value with all of you. You don't have to lose weight just to gain it back and emotionally eat, like I did. You don't have to fail, time and time again. Instead, you can take advantage of the success principles here that will help you build lifelong weight loss and health victories.

So use "Vitamin C" plus the "F-word" together to create your new healthy, healed, and happy lifestyle—one day at a time.

CHAPTER 2

Complete, True Wellness: the Combination and Culmination of the Mind, Body and Soul

"Your mind is your strongest muscle.
The more you use it, the stronger it gets.
So exercise your mind in the most beneficial way.
Don't be your own worst enemy, by allowing it to
be negative. Rather, be your own best friend by
thinking positively and banishing any negative
self talk." —JENNIFER NICOLE LEE

I n today's society, mental illness and negative mindsets are running rampant. Many around us have poisoned minds, from our co-workers to top celebrities, artists, and musicians. Even among those whom our society calls "super-successful people," there are many who are suffering from mental illness, and negative mindsets. Some are dependent upon stimulants and antidepressants just to get them through the day, while others have simply given up and settled for a life filled with negativity, bitterness, and mediocrity. It's sad to see so many on the verge of a nervous breakdown, or a mental meltdown.

But I have great news for you. You don't have to fall victim to the "hungry ghosts" that haunt your mindsets. You can regain control over

42

the most precious domain that has been given to you; your mind. Get ready, because I will show you how to use exercise and eating optimally to help you be more mentally alert, more joyful, have more youthful energy, all while being more focused. This will allow you to really enjoy life to your utmost potential—while leaving all of the mind-draining elements behind.

Clearly, physical fitness isn't the only wellness indicator. Yes, you can get physically fit, but if you don't have the right mental, emotional, and spiritual components woven into your physical fitness, you'll be like a gerbil on a wheel, going nowhere fast. You'll be like I was, on the couch and overweight with no energy, on a rollercoaster ride of emotional and mental ups and downs. It wasn't until I fully realized that in order to enjoy lifelong weight loss and true health, I had to start with my mind, and make it my best friend through positive affirmations, catching all negative self talk, and adjusting my mindset into a much more positive one.

You are equipping your mind with positive ammunition by reading this book. It's a quantum leap in taking the first step to stop failing yourself, by preparing for your healthy lifestyle success. You know by now that you can't get totally healthy with inadequate sleep, eating highly processed foods, and thinking negative thoughts. But that's what many of us do, and don't even realize it. Many people are trying to achieve lifelong weight loss and greater health, but because they are being misled by the diet fluff and "get fit quick" methods, they are not given the tools, tips, and techniques that you have access to with *The Mind, Body & Soul Diet.*

Mental Mindset & Happiness Quiz

We all want to be happy. That's what life is all about. And this is the basis of my Mind, Body and Soul Diet. We have all been on diets before, but the torture, denial, limitations, or sadness that we felt while dieting forced us all to gain the weight back. That is what makes my diet different. It will help you to find your inner happiness and achieve your dream body and perfect fitness level, while relishing your abundantly healthy lifestyle.

Before you go any further, take this quick quiz to rate just how happy you are. For every "yes," give yourself one point.

1. Do you honestly feel that you have full ownership over your happiness?

2. Do you focus on solutions, instead of problems?

3. Do you aim to find the free gifts in life, like in a beautiful sunset?

4. Do you try to make peace with yourself?

5. Do you challenge everything that your mind tells you?

6. When you have bad thoughts, do you question their validity?

7. Do you urge your mind to let go of thoughts that don't serve you?

8. Do you focus on being grateful?

9. Do you practice forgiveness?

10. Do you work to spread loving kindness?

11. Do you nourish your body with super foods, and bountiful nutrition?

12. Do you often tune into your own body's wisdom?

13. Do you feel you are living a life inspired by purpose?

14. Do you follow the inspiration of the moment?

15. Do you feel your life is contributing to something greater than yourself?

16. Do you actively cultivate nourishing relationships?

17. Do you scout out loving, supportive relationships?

18. Are you aware of your own attitude towards life?

19. Do you catch yourself when you become negative, and turn it around?

20. Do you truly believe that thoughts become things?

For every yes, give yourself a point. The more points you have, the more in tune you are with your inner happiness and mental well being. If you have a low score, or want to increase your score, then read on.

So we know that true wellness is a product of three factors: the mind, the body, and finally, the soul. All three are interrelated, integrated and connected. To achieve total wellness and balance, it's essential to address all three areas. And when all three are addressed, your happiness component is increased. You will be happier, or as I like to say, expand your happiness portal. The first component to address is the health of our minds.

As an expert, many have asked me what is the best way to offset mental distress. Certainly, we've all had experience of the many symptoms of mental distress, and they're not fun. Contrary to what other so-called experts state, improving your mental state can be done easily. You don't need to go through endless hours of therapy, and pay those high bills. You can boost your mood and outlook through proper nutrition, eating super foods, enjoying invigorating exercise, and, yes, also by thinking positive thoughts.

If you think you may be suffering from some sort of mental distress, here is a short list to help you identify your feelings:

- Anxiety
- Anger
- Low self-esteem
- Easily agitated
- Easily irritated
- Combative behavior
- Crying often
- Confused thoughts
- Emotional eating
- Unresolved grief issues
- Depression
- Unhealthy thoughts

If you are experiencing any of the symptoms above, my book and I am here to help. I too suffered in my early childhood, in my teenage years, and even in my adulthood, from many of these symptoms—until I took back control over my life and stopped living a life that was less than I deserved. I got off of the wild merry-go-round of emotional instability and the downward spiral of self-inflicted abuse, generated by trying to always please others and not myself, and got on the upward spiral of unlimited health, healing and happiness. Now it's your turn.

I found out the hard way that what we eat and put into our bodies has a direct correlation to our mental well-being. Certain foods, which I call super foods, and which I'll discuss in Chapter 9, can help your mental acuity and give you razor-sharp focus so you won't be distracted by your own mind. You'll be able to make your mind your best friend instead of your worst enemy. In addition to helping you obtain and maintain mental stability and well-being, there is also a visible beauty benefit to eating these super foods. Not only will you be more mentally alert, these foods are also anti-aging, so you will carry your years more gracefully. And the part I love most, and I know that you will too, is that these foods taste absolutely delicious.

There is no doubt that your mind is the most powerful muscle in the body because it directs your entire being, and creates your fate. If you're able to get control of your mind by focusing on what you want to achieve, and not the problems in your life, you will realize your goals. Those who are successful in life don't look left or right, but keep their eyes on the prize. This is a new way of going about life that you must master if you want to make those huge gains and enjoy the blessings that only you can create. Your mind will lead your body and the rest of your life in the right direction. You can easily "train" your mind to be in control. By focusing on only creating prosperity and being positive, this is exactly what you will materialize.

"The first and best victory is to conquer self." —P L A T O

If proper balance is needed to maintain a healthy body, the same is true of our mental state and also our soul. It's amazing that so many timeless insights, from Plato and many other philosophers, are still applicable in today's health field. So read this book with an open mind and true intent to make the necessary improvements.

"Don't aim to change.
Changes can be either good or bad.
But focus on making improvements,
as they are always positive." —JNL

Mary, a single mother of three young children, had gone through a bad divorce and was fired from her job. She had taken many blows in her life, but felt as though she had brought them on herself by letting herself go, and not giving her job the time it needed. She suffered self-inflicted guilt, feeling bad for not being the perfect wife, mother, and employee. She had hit rock-bottom, and didn't know how to pull herself up. I started working with her, rebuilding her inner confidence, helping her re-create her life up from the ashes, and together we made big gains. However, she kept on repeating "JNL, I am going to change, I will change, and I am making changes." This is where her underlying problem was. It was in her belief system that she thought changing was enough. This is not true. In order to make positive results materialize in our lives, we must not merely make changes, but make improvements.

Therefore, don't think of it as making a change, as changes can be either good or bad. Think always of making improvements in your life because improvements are always good. Take a look in your kitchen drawer. Sure, you can change the way it's organized inside, just by shifting its contents around. But it's still just the same old stuff. In order to really improve it, you'll need to toss out utensils that no longer serve you, add a new protective sheet on the bottom, and introduce new tools that will help you to be more efficient and effective.

And speaking of tools, goals are an essential tool that you need to have in your life to make improvements. If you're not waking up and jumping out of bed looking forward to the day, then you don't have enough goals, you don't enough passion, and you don't have enough clarity. I'm going to show you how to make improvements so that your life will be a journey you celebrate every day.

Anticipate Success

"The power of anticipation is what dissects the winners from the losers." —ANTHONY ROBBINS

The number one success principle that separates the failures from the winners, the underachievers from the overachievers, is the power of anticipation. Anticipate success, and you will create it. Anticipate that you will be successful, gain an identity as an athlete, as a super-focused person living a life free of drama, gossip, and negativity. Anticipate that you will live a life full of complete joy, happiness, abundance, prosperity, health, and wealth. Use the power of anticipation, of knowing that you will have a healthier life, and it will happen.

I learned the power of anticipation by observing very successful people. These people projected success into their future, and they didn't let their past failures pull them back or hold them down. I learned how to anticipate the future, and what was going to happen, and then to prepare for my successes. You can also anticipate success by setting goals, both short term and long term, even if you have suffered past failures. By preparing for your success, and anticipating them, you yourself will create your new healthy lifestyle, and achieve your life goals.

"Successful people always bounce back, stronger than before." —JNL

A component to anticipating success is resiliency. Even after you have anticipated your success, obstacles will still come your way, and you must never let them stop you. These roadblocks are simply tests to help us to grow our fortitude and inner strength. We must understand that these obstacles are not permanent, but temporary, and can be overcome by anticipating success, and staying resilient.

I personally have learned the power of being resilient. I was a woman on a mission to finally get rid of my extra eighty-plus pounds. I never gave up or gave in. Like a hacker at a computer, trying to crack the weight loss code, I tried and tried until I got the results I was after. I was persistent and anticipated that I would be successful. Well, it all paid off, because I achieved my own weight loss success, and now I get the joy of helping so many others lose weight for good, and increase the quality of their lifestyles.

"You cannot successfully drive into your future if you are constantly looking in your rear view mirror." —JNL

Letting go of the past is something that we all must learn to do in order to obtain a super healthy, healed and happy lifestyle. When it comes to health and fitness, even top athletes have to be coached through letting go of past defeats and redirecting their focus back to victory. You cannot allow your past failed attempts to cannibalize your soon-successful future. With the Mind, Body and Soul Diet, you will learn how to constructively let go of the past. This will allow you to lose weight, gain muscle, endurance, stamina, and energy while increasing the quality of all areas of your life. By healing yourself, you can become joyful, not jaded, and better, not bitter, and live a sweet life, not a sour one full of pain and resentment. I urge you to realize your true life's potential, and to get out of the passenger seat, and back into the driver seat of your life.

"Failure is just the opportunity to begin again, more intelligently." —HENRY FORD

Part of the Mind, Body and Soul Diet is to have a healthy way to look at our past failures and at failing. We go through some failures so that we can learn. Yes, we are supposed to fail a few times so that we may learn what to do next, and how to go at life better. I would go so far as to say that I have an award in personal failure. I have failed so many times—but I've also learned from my each of my failed attempts. I've learned that, through my belief systems, I can create unsuccessful events in my life or I can create successful ones. What I've learned has enabled me to succeed. And after every past failure, I did get stronger, smarter and better. Let's get real. We all will fail, and there is no sense in beating ourselves up over it. We must fail constructively, learn our lessons, and apply what we learned in our future. It's that simple.

I am not saying that being successful, accomplishing your dream body, or achieving living a super fit life will be easy, but it is worth the journey. Think about the alternatives. Living a life full of stress, struggle, drama, and suffering is not easy either. So you have a choice. And yes, you will be challenged, but this is part of the equation of success.

"A war is raging.
Your mind is the battlefield." —JOYCE MEYER

Remember, it wasn't always easy for me. There was a lot of "inner civil war" in my own mind, and also in my life. We were all raised with some kind of unhealthy belief systems that contradicted what we know to be healthy. Some of mine were:

- Eating a lot of food equals security and safety
- You must please others to be successful
- Being healthy is expensive
- To lose weight, you have to eat "rabbit" food
- Dieting is torture
- Starving yourself is the only way to lose weight
- Cooking healthy takes too much time
- Fast food is easier, quicker, and less expensive
- I am from a heavy-set family, so I will always be fat

I had to learn all over again about food, and how to eat healthy. I also remember that I couldn't make anybody happy. I was too short, too big, too different, not skinny enough, and just plain unpleasing to a lot of people. But the magic and miracles in my life started when I began living my life with self-love and self-respect. I started to please myself first, and lived to make *myself* happy first. That was the real turning point in my life. Slowly but surely, by truly becoming my own best friend, I found that I was allowing those closest to me to be extremely happy and fulfilled, too.

> *"People often say that motivation doesn't last. Well, neither does bathing—that's why we recommend it daily."* —ZIG ZIGLAR

If you are hopeless and need direction, if you've tried in the past, only to fail time and time again, then I am here to tell you that this is a new era for you. Yes, failure is common, but it's not going to be common for you anymore. You have decided to take positive action. The past does not have to equal the future. The countless weight loss success stories from my coaching clients are a result of them anticipating their successes, being resilient, and motivating themselves daily.

In closing, please take a good look below at some of the most successful and important people in history. They did not let their past failures defeat their desires, and they went on to achieve many successes that they were passionate about.

Lucille Ball- Dismissed from drama school with a note that she was wasting her time as she was too shy to put her best foot forward. She went on to be one of the most popular stars world-wide and had one of Hollywood's longest careers.

The Beatles- Turned down by a major recording label because they did not like their sound and "guitar music is on the way out." They went on to be one of, if not the most, revolutionary bands in music history.

Ulysses S. Grant- A failed soldier, failed farmer, and failed real estate agent, who at the age of 38 years old went to go work for his dad as a handy man. He went on to become the 18th President.

Michael Jordan- Cut from the high school basketball team, he went home and locked himself in his room and cried. He is acknowledged by many to be the greatest basketball player of all time.

Thomas Edison- One of his teachers told him that he was too stupid to learn anything, and should go into a field where he would find success by virtue of his pleasant personality. He went on to become one of the most notable American inventors, scientists and businessmen, inventing the light bulb and holding over 1,000 patents.

Walt Disney- Fired from a newspaper because he lacked imagination and had no original ideas. He is a multiple award-winning film producer, director, animator, and innovator in theme park design.

Abraham Lincoln- His fiancé died, he failed in business twice, had a nervous breakdown, and was defeated in 8 elections. He was the 16th President, led America through its greatest internal crisis, and ended slavery.

May these examples encourage you to carry on towards achieving your personal success, even after your failures. Remember, your past does not have to equal your future.

Moments of Enlightenment

I've had many enlightening moments that have led up to my success. These moments were me simply realizing what didn't work, and what did. First of all, I realized that what many women had done in their lives didn't make them happy or fulfilled. Many people, especially women of the past generations, served as sacrificial lambs, so as to speak, for the betterment of their families. They lived to take care of their kids; they lived to put food on the table, always putting themselves last. With my clients, I frequently observed this oxymoron of women working so hard for their families, while silently suffering from bad health and living in misery in their own lives. Their physical, emotional, and mental health suffered greatly, and no one in their family seemed to care. I realized that I was falling into that mold, because I didn't know anything else, and was never shown a better way to live.

When you become a mom—and I know a lot of the mothers out there reading this can relate—your whole identity shifts. Having once felt wanted, desired, and youthful, you begin to feel totally different.

There are times when society doesn't treat you as a whole woman and a beautiful mother, with many wonderful facets. Sometimes it's as if you are looked upon in society as only a baby holder, a baby feeder, and a baby diaper-changer! Your identity as a woman vanishes. It's as if you've become invisible and are only there to serve others and give into other people's needs and desires. And it's especially hard if you don't have a super supportive network of loving friends and family around to help you in your transition into motherhood. It's difficult to put yourself on your own "To-Do List," so you become the last on your list.

This new beginning as a mother was one of my enlightening moments. I realized that not taking time for myself was not healthy. I realized it would end with me being resentful towards my own family, if I did not first take care of myself. I knew that I needed to create time to exercise and prepare healthy meals, not just to sleep all day and eat fast food. I wanted to prove to myself, my family and to society that I could still be a mother and be fit, happy, and fun. I was sick of feeling frazzled and haggard. I yearned to radiate energy that others could sense and see. I wanted to change that paradigm shift, that moms are supposed to be providers and doers for other people all the time around the clock, nonstop, always putting themselves last. Yes, this is an important role as a mother, to nurture and love others, but we must also nurture and love ourselves, a fact we too often overlook

"Put Yourself Back on Your To-Do List." —J N L

This was a positive shift for me. I looked at my own daily to-do list and realized I wasn't on it. Everyone else was on my list. Why wasn't I? I decided then and there to put myself back on my to-do list. I decided to take care of myself, for the betterment of my personal development and growth, and also for the benefit of my family as a whole. I urge you, whether you are a mother, or a busy modern-day woman at the beck and call of many, to start your weight loss journey with self-love and self-respect, by carving out some time in your day to take care of your own well-being.

Take Your Before Photo and Use it As Your Fitness Fuel

Another moment of enlightenment was after the birth of my second son, Dylan. I asked my husband to take a photo of me just to see how I looked. I knew I wasn't healthy. I knew I was out of shape. But, boy was that photo eye-opening! I looked twenty years older than I really was. I had a bleak, drawn-down face, and looked dull, drained, and downright sluggish. Even though my photo was startling, it was one of the most helpful motivators that I could ever have found. I still look at this photo daily to remind me to keep moving forward, and to never allow myself to slip back into unhealthy habits.

I highly recommend that you put down this book and take a "before" photo right now. It's one of the most, important things that you can do, to get you and keep you motivated. Why? It will give you instant clarity. It's like a physical audit. You can see where your body and energy "account" is right now. It will tell you if you need to make "deposits" into your fitness bank account, and to stop making withdrawals.

In order to really see if you are making improvements and prog-ress, you must be able to measure them. Your "before" photo will mark your starting point. It will show where you began. It will represent the beginning of your successful fitness journey. Here comes the fun part. Browse through your favorite fitness or health magazines and choose a photo of someone you would like to look like. Have fun with it! This is the time to celebrate being fit by finding that "after" photo of someone whose body, physique, and inner glow you admire. It will serve as a powerful catalyst, helping you to take positive action to create your own real "after" photo.

"Strong is the new skinny." —JNL

To help me to have a solid future goal in creating the new me, I collected a bunch of "after" photos as well. I had fun breezing through top fitness and health magazines and collecting many different images of strong, fit, healthy, vibrant women who represented the many positive characteristics of what I wanted to become. They were not skinny, but strong. They were not weak, but warriors! And they were not frail looking, but fit.

"In order to take positive action, you must be pushed by a negative, and pulled by a positive." —JNL

So, your "before" photo will be your fitness fuel, pushing you forward, away from your old you. It will push you away from your unhealthy past. Your "after" photo will act as a magnet. It will pull you closer to the new, fit you that you always dreamed of becoming!

"In Sight, In Mind." —JNL

Put your "before" and "after" photos where you can see them daily. I strongly suggest placing them on your vision board. When I started my personal weight loss journey, I put one on my vision board, and then another one in my bathroom where I could see it first thing in the morning. Every day I looked at it and said, "This is the old me. This is the rewind button. I'm not going back here. I love this person and who she is now, but I'm going to get better. I deserve to be healthier and feel physically fit and proud of myself." That's how I lovingly started my complete transformation, leading me to gain my new, improved identity in a spirit of self-love and self-respect. By constantly reminding myself of my personal fitness goals by keeping my "before" and "after" photos in sight, my goals were always foremost in my mind. This technique will definitely help you too.

"Expect More Of Yourself. Raise Your Standards for Yourself."

This simple, yet powerful, exercise helped me to become aware of the self-sabotaging behaviors that were keeping me stuck in a rut. I gave myself a motivational kick in the butt by looking at my "before" photo and saying, "How could I even *live* like this, with such a low level of energy and such a low standard for my body and mind?" This daily exercise helped me to raise my standard of living for myself. Seeing my "before" photo daily made me truly desire a new healthy lifestyle for myself and loved ones. My "before" photo caused me to expect much more of myself and to start creating my new successful future, and your "before" photo will help you to do the same.

At the time, I couldn't stand going to a dressing room; shopping was a complete nightmare. I was stuck in the plus sizes, and I hated bikini season because the first thing I thought about was "What cover-up am I going to wear?" So I started getting really fed up with feeling frustrated, which finally pushed me to expect more out of myself, and raise my standards.

Now, with the Mind, Body and Soul Diet, not only am I at my desired weight, I no longer have to ask myself, "What sarong am I going to wear to the pool?" The only cover-up I ever wear now is sunblock! I said "so long" to my sarong and hello to my new healthy, fit body. With my Mind, Body and Soul Diet principles of self-love and self-respect, not only can I now wear any thing that I want to, but I also have something that can't be bought in a store—which is faith in my own abilities, self confidence, and a winning, "can do" attitude!

I am revealing to you the invaluable lessons that I've learned from my own past mistakes, and from the mistakes of people I've worked from around the world in my coaching consultations. These life lessons will help you to stop sabotaging your own weight loss efforts. You will save time, money, and energy with these personal stories and principles. You will start being instantly more self-reliant and mentally, emotionally, physically, and spiritually stronger.

You will create your own healthy meals, and exercise in the comfort of your own home, or have the confidence to train at your local health club and even take part in a group yoga class. You will start exercising smarter, not harder, to get maximum results in a minimum amount of time in your life. You're going to finally learn what it takes to have lifelong weight loss success. You will also have the tools, tips, and techniques to create success in all areas of your life. Congratulations on your new era.

CHAPTER 3

Diet Secrets Revealed:
Myth Busting

"Don't resolve. Instead, evolve! Let others make their resolutions. They'll only last two weeks. Create your evolution! These improvements will last a lifetime." —JENNIFER NICOLE LEE

In this chapter, I will help you to fully understand what doesn't work and what does, what will give you short-term results, and what will give you long-term results and, lastly, how you can finally stop self-sabotaging behaviors that thwart your success. I've decided to share this message with you because I, too, was lost at one time in the confusing world of fitness. I spent a huge chunk out of my monthly income on an expensive gym membership. I bought prepackaged, cardboard-like, over-processed, and preservative-laden food. I showed up for embarrassing weekly weigh-ins. I hired a glorified "counter" who called himself a trainer, but who always showed up late and checked his cell phone while I worked out. I spent a lot of time, money, and energy trying to get thin. But even at my thinnest, I wasn't happy or fulfilled. I looked at myself in the mirror and said, "I've wanted to be this weight for so long, now I'm finally here, and it's not all it's cracked up to be. I'm still empty inside. I feel lost. I'm still not healed. I still have resentment. I still have not forgiven people in my past—and their memories haunt me daily. And I don't even look healthy, healed, or happy."

It was no wonder that I gained all the weight back, over and over again. I was caught on a self-sabotaging vicious cycle of dieting down only to gain it all back, because I was confused about where to find the keys to lifelong weight loss. I learned the hard way that being able to lose weight forever is so much more than simply the one-dimensional thinking of "calorie in/calorie out." Rather, life-long weight loss success and living a super fit lifestyle is about addressing the mind, body and soul to find true health, healing and happiness.

It pains me to think that I was misled so many times, just like so many other women. I sometimes feel during my consultations with my clients that they must have read my diary from years back! It's like their stories and struggles were mine, too. I'm grateful that I was able to master my health, healing, and happiness through my own *Mind, Body and Soul Diet*. And now I am able to help so many who are in need of solid expert direction. I'm also sad to say that I have consulted with too many people from different backgrounds, of different sizes, with different goals, who have one thing in common: they are silently suffering because of the myths that society has sold them. The are bound by invisible chains of believing that if they eat this and do that that they will be healthy, healed and happy. There is so much more to it! I'm here to banish those myths so you can finally create and embrace your true quality of life.

"Give a man a fish and you feed him for a day. Teach a man to fish and you feed him for a lifetime." —CHINESE PROVERB

Use this section to understand that lifelong success begins with banishing the unhelpful myths that have bound us to our past failures. Gone are the days of you losing weight only to gain it back, or starting to live a healthy lifestyle, only to relapse back to your old unhealthy habits. This is a new era and a new beginning. No more resolutions, because now you are on your evolution!

MYTH 1: ACTIVITY EQUALS RESULTS.

From my extensive experience as a life coach and celebrity trainer, I am perplexed by how many of my clients equate a lot of activity, hard work, struggling, and strain with results. Just because you're moving, doesn't mean you are moving in the right direction or in the right manner. You must know what you want, first of all, to have direction. You must also know the secrets of the ones who have traveled the journey in less time and with less effort so you stay focused and dedicated along the way. I am here to help you get from where you are right now to where you want to be in an easier, simpler, and more enjoyable process than you ever imagined possible.

You don't have to work *harder* to get results. Just work *smarter*. Killing yourself in the gym, beating yourself up mentally with negative self-talk, and eating little to nothing will not get you the results you want. It will only burn you out, and lead you to give up. Rather, being persistent and choosing to be fit one day at a time, plus thinking positively with an "I can do it" attitude, will give you results.

By the same token, people try the boot camp, drill-sergeant workout routine because they think they have to punish themselves into getting results. Being healthy is not about punishment. It's about giving fresh blood and oxygen to all the cells of your body. It's about eating optimally to boost your mental acuity, blast fat, tone muscle, and balance your emotions. Being healthy makes you happier while you're losing weight and building endurance and stamina, as well as sleek and sexy muscle tone. And you won't lose weight by torturing yourself with difficult-to-do exercises which may actually cause you injury, thus placing you further away from your weight loss goals.

So many people aren't seeing the results they want because they're still living life with the outdated and unhelpful belief system that the harder they work, the more results they'll get. I want you to embrace the new success principle of the Mind, Body and Soul Diet.

Truth: It's about working smarter, not harder, to get maximum results in minimum time, while making it fun and enjoying the process. The smarter you work, the more results you will get—and most importantly you will enjoy it and stick with your new healthy lifestyle.

MYTH 2: BY DOING THE SAME THING, YOU WILL GET DIFFERENT RESULTS.

If you've tried many times to lose weight but have failed, that simply goes to show that what you've done in the past doesn't work. Einstein said, "Insanity is doing the same thing over and over again and expecting different results." This saying is and will always be true. And that's why you've not been seeing the results you desire, because you've kept on doing the same thing over and over again, expecting a different result. Remember what I said before; you can't use your rearview mirror to help you steer toward your future.

I congratulate you for reading this book, because now you're going to let go of the past while embracing the future so you may progress. Now you'll develop a new belief system, letting go of the false information that has hindered you, while embracing the Mind, Body and

Soul Diet success principles. So congratulations, you're on your way to lifelong success!

Truth: When old methods don't work, seek out new and improved ways to get healthy. Be open to the new principles in this book, and be ready for the improvements in your life.

MYTH 3: ANYONE CAN HELP YOU LOSE WEIGHT.

Many people with great intentions of getting healthier listen to so-called fitness experts or gurus who have not personally gone through a weight loss transformation before. Some sadly even lean on their friends and family who have little to no experience in the field. Choose your life coach and trainer very carefully. I like to say that information and expertise are power. Don't waste your time trying to follow some novice's advice, or leaning onto a friend or family member who doesn't share your fitness goals. This could actually be dangerous, as the science of weight loss is not their expertise.

Truth: Rather, find someone who has gotten the results that you want and see what they've done. I myself have lost over eighty pounds by following my own Mind, Body and Soul Diet principles. I know what it's like to be a woman wearing five different hats at once: mom, wife, life coach, entrepreneur, and CEO of my own company. I know what it's like to multitask and still have to get the results that I want. It's my passion to empower and help others who want to create the same success in their lives.

"Success leaves clues," I always say. Stop following so-called fitness experts who don't have that reliability factor, who haven't experienced that journey for themselves. When I began my weight loss journey, it was hard for me to even listen to others who were always in shape, or fit, and who had never been overweight or gone through being pregnant. I know first-hand what it is like to be over 200 pounds, to be pregnant, and to breastfeed during those sleepless nights. But I did it! And if I can do it, so can you.

I'm still on the journey, and I'm going to show you how to join me on the right path. I am always here to listen and coach you one-on-one. You can apply for a personal, private one-on-one life coaching consultation with me at www.ClubJNL.com.

MYTH 4: A CALORIE-IN, CALORIE-OUT FORMULA EQUALS WEIGHT LOSS SUCCESS.

So many people think it's about just cutting back their calories while increasing exercise. Yes, the results may come, but they will only be temporary… I'll say it as many times as I have to: to enjoy weight loss success, you must include the mind, the body, and the soul.

Truth: To achieve lifelong, everlasting weight loss and optimal health means so much more than just what you put into your mouth. It's also the thoughts and ideas that you put into your head. Start tapping into your mental strength. Understand how important both mental well-being and mastery over your emotions are. Increasing the quality of your spirituality will complete your foundation, not only in helping you to lose weight but also improving all areas of your life. For example, you can eat 1,600 calories per day of sugar-coated cereal, and exercise only doing cardio. Yes, you will lose weight. However, you can also eat 1,800 (yes 200 calories more) of mind-boosting foods, chock full of antioxidants, vitamin, and minerals—and lose weight! And you can enjoy a variety of exercises such as meditation, yoga, and cardio which also tighten and tone your muscles. The latter of these two diet plans will help you reach your goals, while helping you to increase your health, heal you, and also make you happier.

MYTH 5: LOSING WEIGHT AND GETTING HEALTHY ISN'T FUN.

Almost everyone I talk to thinks that in order to lose weight they have to endure pain and punishment. Why lose weight if you're not going to enjoy it? It's not boring or painful. It isn't punishment.

In my coaching sessions, I help recondition and retrain my fitness friends to look at living a healthy lifestyle as fun. Try shifting your mindset from "I *have* to workout" to "I *get* to workout!" You will instantly see how beneficial exercising is to you, and that it's nothing to be loathed, but ought to be celebrated. You get to give fresh blood and oxygen to all the cells in your body. You get to have that one hour of special "me" time—away from everybody else—when you're connecting with your Higher Power and engaging in positive self-talk. You get to stop being seduced by other people's distractions and urgencies and lives. Exercise is a gift you give yourself!

Do this important activity daily. Ask yourself this very empowering question: How can I gain stamina, endurance, and energy and enjoy the process and have fun doing it? Your mind will give you the answers. Remember, your mind is a brilliant creation. If you ask it questions, it will answer you honestly and help you. For instance, when you ask yourself "How can I lose weight and make it fun?," you may decide one day to finally try that kick-boxing class you've always wanted to check out. The next day you may want to go bike riding, and the next day enjoy a brisk power walk. You see, being physically fit is not as boring or as cookie-cutter as we have been led to believe. So ask yourself this question each and every day and you will see that you enjoy the journey to getting the results you want.

Truth: Exercise is the greatest gift you can give yourself. Exercising is fun!

MYTH 6: LOSING WEIGHT HAS TO HAPPEN NOW!

People sabotage themselves all the time because they are suffering from either "I-want-it-now-itis" or "Get-there-now-itis." This is my "medical" scientific terminology for when people demand and expect results now. This is the worst kind of self-sabotaging behavior, because when weight loss doesn't happen fast enough, they get discouraged and give up.

Here is my own story of how I almost threw in the towel and gave up. After two and a half months of my weight loss and transformational program, I still hadn't seen the results I wanted, even though I was working out about 5 days a week and eating healthy every day. I was at a crossroads, and I was about to quit. I mean, almost three months and no results? Come on? I was at the end of my rope!

Before I gave up and gave in, I remember thinking that even if my weight on the scale didn't budge or that I hadn't dropped any clothes sizes yet, that I was still practicing healthy habits. I was proud of myself for exercising and eating healthy. That was the magic: me being proud of me for being healthy, and not so caught up with the scale. So I decided just to keep at it and not to stress myself over the scale or my clothes size. Then it happened.

I let go of having to see results immediately. Once I released my need for instant gratification, the weight started melting off. For me, this came at around the third month. I'm so glad now that I didn't give up when I was tempted. That's why I'm here to tell you, never give up.

Truth: Don't expect results overnight. Go back to Myth 5 and realize you can enjoy the journey. Give yourself the gift of time. Don't throw in the towel after two weeks. It's not a New Year's resolution. It's a complete evolution! You're in an evolutionary stage, and you're going to evolve into a new, better, healthier, whole, healed you. Remember the saying "Rome wasn't built in a day." Understand that you are a masterpiece in the making, a work in progress, so give yourself the time to evolve into your new improved you!

MYTH 7: YOU MUST SERIOUSLY RESTRICT YOUR CALORIES TO LOSE WEIGHT

We all have been there. Okay—it's Monday—it's diet time—so we cut back on calories. But by 5:00 in the afternoon, we are eating the paint off of the walls! We suffer from the "I've-been-good-all-day-itis," eating nothing all day, only to be starving by the end of the day.

Look at it this way. How do farmers fatten a pig? The same exact way many of us have fattened ourselves; by not eating all day, and then eating a huge dinner at night. Farmers intentionally fatten up pigs by not feeding them much during the day, getting the pigs really hungry and building up their appetites, so that when they're finally fed, they want to binge. Then they feed them as much slop as they want, allowing the pigs to eat for as long as they want, so that they'll gorge themselves. Not feeding the pig much during the day slows down the pig's metabolism, thus making it hold onto fat—not exactly what we want to be doing in our quest to lose weight!

Here is another powerful analogy: How does a tiny Japanese baby become a gigantic Sumo wrestler? Again, just like the farmer's pig, he doesn't eat all day long while he's doing rigorous grappling and wrestling exercises. Then he sits down for a three- or four-hour meal with endless portions.

That's exactly what I did during my yo-yo dieting phase, and it's the same thing many of you are doing right now. You don't eat all day long, and then you're so hungry when you get home you'll eat the paint off the wall. I want you to reverse that. Eat breakfast like a queen, eat lunch like a princess, and eat dinner like a pauper. That way you are trickling down your calories from the rest of the day. Working with your metabolism, not against it, by eating more calories earlier in the day rather than later, is what will give you weight loss success.

Truth: Aim to eat 5 to 6 meals a day, to keep yourself fueled and your energy up. Work with your metabolism and not against it, by eating every 2 to 3 hours.

CHAPTER 4

The Mind, Body & Soul Diet

"What makes a precious diamond so rare? Its delicate intricacies and depth. Just like a diamond, your life has many dimensions that add up to ultimate quality of life. Embrace and nurture your mind, your body, and your soul, for whole balance and complete wellness that will radiate brilliance —just like the diamond." —JENNIFER NICOLE LEE

I n this chapter I will introduce the complete Mind, Body and Soul Diet to give you optimal health in all areas of your life. No longer will you be happy in one area of your life and not in another. This is about creating balance, wholeness, and wellness; it's about being centered in your own life, now and forever—just like a flawless diamond with many sides, cuts, and dimensions.

As I briefly explain the three components of this diet, observe how they build on each other for maximum results. We will then explore each component in more depth in its own chapter. In the next chapter, I will focus on the power of your mind. I will show you how to have it work for you, instead of against you.

The Mind

"Whether you believe that you can or you can't, you are right." —HENRY FORD

"Every thought has the power to either wound or to heal." —DEEPAK CHOPRA

This is the first most important component of the Mind, Body and Soul Diet. Your mind is your strongest muscle. Whatever you put into your mind will trickle down to your body. If you are able to understand that you must be on a diet free of negative self-talk and negative mental energies that keep you blocked and locked into where you are, you will be able to harness the power of your mind.

Remember, we live in a society in which instant gratification is highly prized. We want to be healed, now. We want to be skinny, now. We want to be fit, now. We want everything overnight. If anything takes three seconds longer than expected, we get peeved.

Part of building mental strength is the understanding that reaching your goals will not happen in a blink of an eye. Only with persistence and determination will you get results. So stop trying to be perfect, living by that black and white, all-or-nothing mentality.

"Boy, does that lady look so sexy, happy and fit. I hate her." —ANONYMOUS

Not everyone in your life will be happy when you start losing weight, feeling great, and radiating positive energy. You cannot let these negative influences—I call these pesky "energy vampires"—steal your motivation. It's just another opportunity for you to cut yourself free of anchors that are holding you back and down.

I experienced backlash from others who weren't so happy when I started to unzip and melt off my fat suit. They talked behind my back and were secretly jealous. It's hard to believe that not everyone would be happy when you finally crack your weight loss code, and start melting off the pounds. When I finally started detoxing my life, eliminating the toxins, it seems like my toxic so-called "friendships" started to eliminate themselves too.

So what did I do? Cry over it? Get upset about not everyone being happy that I was finally able to achieve my dream body? No way! This was the most cleansing time of my life. I became free from binding, poisonous relationships that no longer served me. Hanging out with those who did not support my dreams or goals was something that I no longer could even fathom doing. I had built up too much inner strength, confidence, power, self-love, and self-respect to even consider it.

As you're shedding your fat suit, you will also be shedding old, outdated behaviors that no longer serve you. Say goodbye to empty, and say hello to being empowered!

Here are some exercises that you can do, to help get you and keep you empowered:

- Banish all jealous, negative, hurtful, vindictive people from your inner circle.
- Tell yourself that you can and you will.
- Think healing thoughts, not harmful thoughts.
- Write your to-do list the night before, to keep focused.

- Ask yourself what you should be focusing on right now, so you stay aligned with your goals.

- Harness the power of visualization. If Olympic gold medalists and NASA astronauts can use the power of visualization to mentally walk themselves through some of the most challenging situations in their lives, there's no reason you can't as well.

- Create a vision board, and put your dream body on it next to your "before" photo.

- Pick out a photo of someone you hold in high regard and also put him or her on your vision board.

- Be eager to trade hours of unnecessary cardio with only a small amount of time at weight training, to get amazing body-shaping and strength-conditioning results, which will also boost your energy instead of depleting it.

- When you start losing weight and feeling great, don't get scared and sabotage your own results, thus forcing you back to your starting point. Rather, embrace and welcome the positive changes in your life.

- Meditate daily, even if it is only for five minutes, to reflect on your personal goals.

Your level of mental strength and mental fortitude is also directly correlated to what you put into your body. Eating the superfoods I'll tell you about in Chapter 9 will help boost your mental facility and productivity. I've seen so many "physically fit" people who are mentally "soft." They allow failures to rule their lives, and keep them locked where they are. A big part of the problem is that they are not eating the right foods, which their brains actually need to function at their best. Food, as well as physical and mental exercises, can help boost your mental acuity and increase your ability to focus and be more aware.

In Chapter 5 where I address the mind, I'll help you to learn how to no longer be ruled by your emotions but instead to learn true self-mastery.

The Body

"The body is a sacred temple;
treat it as such." —JENNIFER NICOLE LEE

Your body is, of course, the one and only body you will ever have. Treat it with respect and it will perform better, and you will be stronger and fitter. Think of it this way—you have the decision to go through this life with an energy level of, say, a 1975 Volkswagen Bug putt-putting along, or the energy of a sleek and sexy new 500-plus horsepower Ferrari, with endless energy and drive. It's your choice. You can fill yourself with unleaded gasoline or premium fuel.

Consider this analogy. Would you give your best friend whom you love dearly a fat-laden, artery-clogging cheeseburger with deep-fried, gut-bloating french fries? Or would you give her a crisp, fresh garden salad topped with grilled salmon, loaded with essential fatty acids, which her body needs and craves? Of course you would give her the salad! So why don't you do this for yourself?

In order for you to want to put healthy, nutrient-dense food into your body, you must view your body as a temple. It is a matter of self-respect. It's not about starving and eating pre-packaged diet food.

Rather, it's about eating healthy foods that are nutrient-dense and give you the greatest energy, the best fuel, and the highest stamina level.

Many use the excuse not to eat healthy food by choosing to believe that it is too expensive or that it takes too much time to prepare. This belief could not be further from the truth. It's a cinch to go grocery shopping once a week, and get fresh fruits and vegetables, raw nuts, and lean meats that are rich in protein. Also, now the fast food industry is wising up, thanks to our demands for healthier food choices. Many, if not all, of the major fast food chains are offering fresh salads topped with grilled chicken, fruit cups, and also lighter or reduced-calorie fare. So remember, your body is a sacred living creation, and it deserves the best food and nutrients you can give it.

"Balance from within, equals tranquility out." —J N L

"There is such a thing as overtraining. You are not getting to your fitness goals faster by overtraining, but actually slowing down the process." —J N L

Working out must also incorporate balance. Replace the energy you expend with rest. Banish the thinking that the more you train, the more results you will get. Overtraining doesn't help anyone.

If you think you may be overtraining, here are some telltale signs:

- Washed-out feeling; tired, drained or lack of energy
- Moodiness and irritability
- Depression

- Loss of enthusiasm for the sport

- Increased incidence of injuries

- Insomnia

- Headaches

If you have several of these overtraining symptoms, the best thing to do is to look at how many times you are training in a week. You should aim to train no less than 3 times per week, to no more than 5 or 6 times per week. Again, it's important to understand that fitness is a lifelong journey to be enjoyed, and not a one-time event. Also, you must give your mind, body and soul a much-needed break if you've been overtraining.

One of my clients, Sara, was a diehard fitness fanatic who never missed her twice-a-day workouts. She confided to me that she always felt lethargic, and that she had missed her period a time or two. She looked drawn in the face, and didn't radiate that inner glow of health. She had also started to feel as if her body was breaking down, or getting beat up. I asked her to take a serious look at her exercise program. She trained seven days a week, and felt guilty if she missed a workout. The funny part is that she had hit a plateau and stopped losing weight. She actually started gaining it back. Obviously, what she was doing was not helping her, but hindering her. She sought me out for much-needed expert help.

I had to coach and consult with her a lot to get her down to training four days a week, with a fifth day allotted for an active mediation and or a yoga session to help balance her body again and regain the stamina and tranquility that she needed. What I also noticed from analyzing her lifestyle was that she didn't make time for any anti-aging, re-energizing beauty rituals, such as a massage, an Epsom salt bath (to mineralize the body) or a facial.

So I helped her to counteract her overtraining by actually scheduling in days of rest, and also at-home spa treatments. This helped her to regain the balance in her life. And the best part was that the goal for weight loss that she'd had in the first place, started to happen. Sara thanked me for helping her to "take one step back to take ten steps ahead." She now had enough energy to train efficiently. The secret lay in getting in enough rest.

There are many ways in which you can give yourself the necessary rest. This can be accomplished by meditating, relaxing, and creating beauty rituals. These balancing practices are not luxuries, but essential. Have you ever seen people who lose weight, only to wind up looking exhausted, with dry skin and pale, drawn faces that don't radiate health? This is due to overtraining and not taking part in anti-aging, beautifying rituals. Warm baths, spa treatments, facials, and massages may sound indulgent, but they are necessary practices that put energy back into your body. They are investments in your overall health. As you do them, you are putting much-needed deposits back into your depleted energy resources and your body.

JNL-Approved At Home Spa Treatments

Here are some of my favorite at-home spa treatments you can indulge in on any budget, and work into your busy schedule. Stop denying yourself a healthy lifestyle and take positive action. Be willing and brave enough to start a brand-new, fresh path towards your ultimate fitness level and healthy lifestyle. Practice a little much-needed self-love in allowing yourself to enjoy one of these simple spa treatments, which you can do in the comfort of your own home:

EPSOM SALTS BATHS:

Epsom Salt has dozens of healthful benefits. Using Epsom Salt is a natural way to relax the nervous system, treat skin problems, and draw toxins from the body. This long-time remedy has been useful for almost everything from aching limbs, back pain, healing cuts, muscle strain, colds and congestion, soreness from childbirth, and flushing toxins and heavy metals from the body. The magnesium sulfate of Epsom Salt acts as a muscle relaxant, and by easing muscle pain it helps the body to eliminate harmful substances.

If your goal is to combat stress, then taking a dip in an Epsom Salt bath is essential! Stress can drain magnesium, a natural stress-reliever, from the body. Magnesium is necessary for the body to bind adequate amounts of serotonin, a mood-elevating chemical within the brain that creates a feeling of calm and relaxation.

Feet aching? Then soak those tired feet in a pan of water with half a cup of Epsom Salt. This will not only make your feet feel better. The added benefit is that they'll smell better too. Epsom Salt neutralizes odors and softens skin. If you suffer from dry, flaky skin, then try rubbing Epsom Salt directly on the body, as it exfoliates skin and leaves it smooth and silky. You can add essential oils or mix with baby oil. Keep some of this mixture by the sink if you wash your hands a lot. The combination can help treat dry skin problems.

GREEN TEA FOOT BATHS:

After a long day, your legs and feet can feel hot and achy. For fast relief, dip your feet in iced green tea. According to Chinese medicine, it's considered a cooling tea that absorbs body heat, leaving you feeling refreshed in minutes.

MILK BATHS:

Milk baths strewn with rose petals worked for Cleopatra, and there's no reason that it will not do the same for you. Mix half cup of milk powder with your bath water and see the difference.

RED DESERT CLAY BATHS:

Red desert bathing clay is an excellent way to gently detox your entire body. Its ionic charge is so strong that it draws out many toxins through the skin. It's something that I highly recommend, as it's powerful yet relaxing, and soft on your body. Try the Red Desert Bathing Clay from www.i-amperfectlyhealthy.com.

COLLAGEN-BOOSTED DRINKS:

If you want to turn back the clock, then add a scoop of collagen powder to your drinks. Originally studied in Japan for their ability to improve joint health, beverages infused with collagen powder turned out to have an unexpected bonus: every single person who used them reported gaining firmer, clearer, smoother skin, stronger nails, and softer, fuller hair. Try Neocell Labs Super Collagen Powder.

MASSAGE AWAY EYE PUFFINESS:

If your eyes look puffy, it could be because excess fluid accumulates in the area overnight. Want a quick fix? Dab a little of your favorite eye cream onto your two ring fingers and gently massage your eye area, moving from the inner corner to the temple. Repeat four to six times.

DEBLOAT AND DEPUFF IN MINUTES:

Suffering from a heavy sodium meal the night before, and feeling bloated in the belly and puffy in the face? Try 3 minutes on the Ab Circle Pro. It's one of the most effective pieces of exercise equipment that I have ever tried. It helps to get fresh blood and oxygen to your face within seconds, and also to tighten and tone up your tummy. After 3 minutes, I feel like I am wearing an invisible corset!

DRY HANDS:

We all have to wash the dishes, right? For a quick hydrating treatment for your hands while doing your dishes, cover your hands with a thick layer of lotion and wear latex cleaning gloves. The warm dishwater helps you to get the deep lotion treatment, while the gloves provide insulation for the heat.

"SWEET AS HONEY" FACIAL:

To keep your face naturally beautiful and free of any common skin problems, splash your face with warm water and massage it with a tablespoon of honey. Honey is naturally antibacterial, so it will help to fight off any blemishes on the rise. Splash your face well afterwards with warm water. You can also use plain yogurt instead of honey, which works as an exfoliant, as its lactic acid dissolves dead skin cells.

As you can see, at-home beauty is yours for pennies a day, while making huge deposits in your well-being.

For more at home *Mind, Body and Soul Diet* beauty spa treatments, visit www.MindBodyandSoulDiet.com

The Soul

"Man cannot live by bread alone." —JESUS CHRIST

We must be spiritually fed to fully enjoy life to its utmost potential. We can survive on physical nutrients alone; however, life would be very dull and unfulfilling. When we're down and out, when we've had a bad day, when nothing seems to be going right, and life is coming at us from all angles, this is when spiritual practice comes into play.

CHANGES: Life/ Outerworld/ No Control Over

CONSTANT: You/ Innerworld/ What you can Directly Control

EXAMPLE: Fired/ Breakup/ Death

Exercise + Eat for optimal Health

This illustration above shows you how you can set your life up for success, and make the conscious decision to stay focused on your lifestyle goals, even when life happens. The common denominator at the bottom of this equation is eating and exercising for optimal health. That never changes. And on top of that equation is life. Life is going to happen to you. You may have a bad day, get into a tiff with a loved one, or maybe even get laid off. However, even in life's darkest and loneliest times, you must still take care of yourself by exercising and eating for optimal health.

What must never change is your common denominator in life. Even when your life isn't turning out the way you want it to, and you are challenged daily, you must still work out and eat right. This new, healthy habit will help you in dealing with all of life's obstacles. Even though life changes and frustrates you, you must never steer away from your improved program. Through practicing this Mind, Body and Soul Diet principle of choosing to exercise and eat healthy, nutrient-dense meals, you'll be that much more successful in all areas of your life. That's why your spiritual health is so important to keep you going. It's your fuel to keep you motivated and inspired to never give up or give in. In Chapter 7: The Soul, I'll share with you techniques to keep you headed in the right direction, no matter what life throws your way.

The Whole Is Greater than the Sum of the Parts

You are a complete, whole individual. Your Creator made you this way. That means you are not just your body. You are a complex being made up of mental, emotional, and spiritual components. If you are off balance, it will show up in your body and in your health. You are probably overeating because something is bothering you emotionally. Or there's pain in your life, and you seek out comfort from food. Perhaps a negative memory keeps haunting you. Don't allow your past bleak experiences to bleed over and taint your future. Remember, your past does not equal your future. From your new healthy habits, you will be creating a new, better life for you and your loved ones. Aim to be whole again, by allowing a new, improved, better way of living to work miracles in your life. Use the F-word—faith—plus Vitamin C—confidence—to yield positive results in your life.

It's plain to see that focusing on just one area of your life doesn't work in creating true balance and overall health. Can going the one-dimensional approach provide any relief? Sure, but it's a quick fix, or what I call a band-aid approach, and it's short-term at best. Your problem may be fixed temporarily because something is covering it up, but you haven't addressed it from the root. Say that you are suffering emotionally from a bad experience, but you are still exercising. You must take the time to heal yourself emotionally to insure you don't let it put you off balance, or negatively impact other areas of your success. It's what you've probably been doing up until now, and you know as well as I do that, if it works at all, it only lasts a short time.

"The truth shall set you free." —JOHN 8:32

You may lose weight, but if your emotions are not in check, then you will only gain it back. If your career is doing great, but you are not exercising and eating right, then you are still off balance. Look at your life and see what needs to be addressed the most. Be honest and true to yourself and you will live a healthier, healed, happier life.

This doesn't mean that you can't focus on one area in which you're weaker than in others. Working on the area of mental health and mastering your emotional states, for example, makes weight loss that much easier. It will help you not to eat emotionally, the most common reason for obesity. Working on your spiritual health will make you strong enough to work out even on those hard days that you just don't want to exercise. I personally rely on my spiritual strength, when my body is tired and I feel like I don't have the energy to workout. When I lean on my spirituality, I rediscover the strength I need to start my workouts and finish them.

The central message behind *The Mind, Body & Soul Diet* is to heal ourselves fully and completely, instead of putting that instant, quick fix band-aid on our problems and covering them up. When you heal every area of your life and let go of the past—memories, emotions, habits, paradigms, mindsets and attitudes that no longer work for you—you actually create room for new blessings: blessings of health and mental peace, blessings of being able to control your emotional state to create balance in your life, and blessings of positive attitudes and habits, which will make it possible to create your dream body.

CHAPTER 5

The Mind

"The mind is the strongest muscle of the body. The more you use it, the stronger it gets. It has the power to create and to destroy; it can be your worst enemy or your best friend. I'm going to teach you how to make it your best friend, by having it work for you, not against you!" —JENNIFER NICOLE LEE

Your mind is one of the greatest and most powerful gifts that you have been given. But many people sabotage this power by living in constant mental civil war—and they don't even know it. They're holding on to archaic, outdated belief systems, while hoping for a better outcome. Little do they know that their belief systems subconsciously prevent their dreams and goals from materializing in their lives.

The Mind, Body and Soul Diet identifies how mental health and self-mastery will help you stop suffering from what I call approach/avoidance. Approach/avoidance occurs when you start creating success in your life, then suddenly you get scared. You start getting comments from other people that make you uncomfortable, so you shrink back into your old self. Or you start slipping back on taking action toward your goals; for instance, you go and get fast food instead of doing your weekly grocery shopping for healthy meals.

Mental clarity is priceless, especially in today's information age, when we are bombarded with information every split second from every direction. We must constantly guard how we use our minds, what we decided to focus on or to think about. We must also be diligent in questioning all of our thoughts. As the author Joyce Meyer insightfully wrote, "There is a war raging and your mind is the battlefield."

One way of gaining control of your mind and harnessing the power of your focus is to know exactly what it is you want, with clarity and conviction. I've heard so many times in my weight loss clients' consultations about what they don't want. For example, I always hear: "I'm tired of having no energy; I'm sick of looking this way; I don't want to be in a size 16 the rest of my life." Remember the Mind, Body and Soul Diet principle that you get more of what you focus on? So, if you are focusing on what you don't want, then that is exactly what you will get more of.

> *"The more you talk about what you don't want, or talk about how bad it is—well, you are creating more of that."* —JACK CANFIELD in *The Secret*

Right now, you're probably focusing on what you don't want and talking about it, and this is undoubtedly part of the reason why you are not getting the results that you desire. It's a law of metaphysics: what you focus on, you will create more of. What you focus on will actually manifest in your life. In essence, to manifest means to make your thoughts reality. So use the power of focus to create a healthier you. If you believe you will get healthier every day, then you will. But, you must be clear in your focus. In this chapter, you will learn how to gain clarity, how to make goal-setting easy, how to stop self-sabotaging behaviors, and how to stop the mental "civil war" that only confuses and frustrates you.

It's been scientifically proven that we human beings only use about ten percent of our brains. Just think of what we could accomplish if we used more of our brain power and our ability to zero in on what counts. Many of us find it hard to focus on what we should be focusing on. This lack of positive focus is caused by us being constantly distracted by other people's wants and desires, seduced by the notion that the more we multitask and do, the more important we are.

At one time, I didn't know what I wanted to do, or what I wanted to be, or even what my fitness and life goals were. I discovered for myself the priceless tools of harnessing the power of focus, and gaining clarity with simple goal-setting. I will help you to stop being confused and to gain the power of focus and clarity so that you too can carve out your life's goals and passions.

"Use the power of questions to help you achieve your goals in life." —ANTHONY ROBBINS

I have figured out how to keep my mental focus and acuity with the tools, tips, and techniques below. These are the questions that I ask my coaching clients and myself to help gain clarity and cut out the clutter, thus redirecting the focus on what really matters.

QUESTIONS TO ASK TO GAIN CLARITY AND FOCUS:

1. What do I want?
2. Why do I want it?
3. How will I achieve it?

4. What's holding me from achieving these goals?

5. How can I get around what's hindering me from achieving my goals?

6. What is the purpose of achieving this goal?

7. Who can help me achieve my goals?

8. Who has already done what I want to achieve? What can I learn from them?

9. Who are really my true friends, who want to help me achieve my goals?

10. Does this thought, thing, or person help me in achieving my goals, or hinder me?

These questions have helped me to stop riding the fence of indecision. I urge you too to stop the do-si-do of going one step forward and one step back. This is the pattern of approach/avoidance in which you expend a lot of energy, but go nowhere. I too suffered from wanting to lose weight, but failing to take action, not wanting to get up and go to the gym. I gained the super-focused mental vision and started making my mind work for me and not against me. I urge you to do the same.

Mind, Body and Soul Tools, Tips, and Techniques

"The secret of success is learning how to use pain and pleasure instead of having pain and pleasure use you. If you do that, you're in control of your life. If you don't, life controls you." —TONY ROBBINS

TIP #1: USE THE PAIN VERSUS PLEASURE PRINCIPLE.

We are driven by two distinct sensations: pain and pleasure. Our actions are always based upon moving towards pleasure and away from pain. These two pillars of pain and pleasure really create our behaviors. If you haven't lost weight, or you've lost weight only to gain it back, you are probably linking more pain to working out and eating optimally, and more pleasure to not working out and not eating healthy.

I've had a lot of people tell me, "JNL, if I lose weight, my best friend will be jealous;" or "Losing weight means I have to starve myself and exercise obsessively." One client of mine once said, "If I lose weight, I'll just have saggy skin and I won't look attractive anyway." Another didn't want to work out because it meant she couldn't spend quality time with her family. Their excuses showed me that these women had linked pain to exercising and eating right…

These are examples of self-sabotaging beliefs that equate working out, losing weight, and getting healthy with pain instead of pleasure. These people have actually struck out before getting up to bat. They are still struggling in their own self-inflicted mental "civil war." They are more in love with their excuses than they are with their goals. Don't fall into the same trap of playing the victim. Instead, plot and prepare for your success, and become victorious by finding and creating ways to weave new, healthy habits into your life that will stick.

MIND, BODY AND SOUL DIET EXERCISE: LINK PAIN TO NOT BEING HEALTHY AND PLEASURE TO BEING HEALTHY

Let's flip this mentality and mindset of linking pain to a healthy lifestyle on its head. I want you to start linking pain to not working out, to not losing weight, to not eating optimally, simply by looking one year ahead.

Ask yourself, "Where will I be if I don't start exercising and eating optimally?" Will you be twenty, thirty, fifty, or even sixty more pounds overweight? And where would you start then? Start linking real pain to not being able to wear the things you want to wear, not having a higher energy level, or just feeling and looking older than you probably are right now. Link more pain to that "before" photo you took. Link pain to the frustration you feel at going through life with low self-esteem, not being able to do the things you want to do, and not having the energy to get up and achieve your goals.

Now, here comes the fun part. Start linking pleasure to working out and eating optimally. Tell yourself that by exercising you are giving yourself the gift of fresh blood and oxygen to all of the cells in your body. By choosing health-boosting foods, you are giving your body and mind the fuel they need to achieve all your goals and do the things you love, like spending time with your family or pursuing a new career, or beginning a hobby you have always wanted to try. This tool will help you take action in your life and in your mind.

TIP #2: MAKE YOUR MIND YOUR BEST FRIEND.

"I'm nice to people who are mean to me. And I am mean to myself, when I should be nice. This is the definition of insanity." —ANONYMOUS

On the whole, people beat themselves up. We drive ourselves crazy with shame, guilt, self-inflicted judgments and not feeling as though we're good enough. We forget that it's not about being perfect; it's about being persistent.

So what if you missed a workout this week? So what if you went on a cruise and gained five pounds? Don't fall victim to overwhelming yourself with negative self-talk by calling yourself a fat pig. Just understand that you are human and give yourself the gift of time to get in shape.

Mind, Body and Soul Diet Exercise: Ban All Guilt, Blame, and Shame, and Zap all Negative Self-Talk Right When It Starts.

Now is the time to become aware of that little destructive voice inside your head that creeps up once in a while. Tell that little negative inner voice and self-sabotaging alter ego exactly who is in control and who is the boss; you! One way I stop unconstructive, negative self-talk right in its tracks is by acknowledging it right when it starts and then flipping that comment right on its head. It's a Mind, Body and Soul Diet principle that works wonders. As soon as you hear, "I will never lose this weight," flip it into something positive and repeat it to yourself at least three times. Tell yourself, "I will and can lose this weight, and I will make it fun and enjoyable. It won't happen overnight, but it will happen with me being persistent, and not focusing on being perfect."

Here is another Mind, Body and Soul Diet technique. Instantly zap any and all negativity by looking at your past victories, no matter how big or small they are. Remember when you got to your training on time? Remember when you chose that protein shake over that candy bar? Remember when you walked into that sculpting class for the first time? You have many achievements and accomplishments that you should be proud of, so reflect upon them to give yourself an instant jolt of positivity.

Another Mind, Body and Soul Diet technique is to use the power of questions. Ask yourself empowering questions like: How can I make exercising fun? How can I really gain control over my mind? What do I need to be focusing on right now? How can I learn more about brain-boosting foods that can help me to gain clarity in my life? Your mind will give you answers, and you will reawaken, recharge, and re-motivate your mind, body and soul!

TIP #3: MIND, BODY AND SOUL GOAL SETTING MADE SIMPLE.

Too many people are mentally bogged down in other people's to-do lists, other people's emergencies, other people's urgencies, and other people's expectations. Here is my Mind, Body and Soul method for getting rid of the mental clutter, getting real with yourself, and gaining clarity through three empowering and enlightening questions.

Step 1: Ask Yourself, *"What Do I Really Want?"* Ask yourself with brutal honesty what you really, really want. Take this moment to be truly free in expressing your desires and wishes. Allow yourself to dream, and dream big, when asking yourself what your goals are. What do you want your physical fitness level to be? What do you want to achieve in your life? What would you like to accomplish professionally? What do you want to achieve for your family? This step lays the foundation of your goal-making process.

Step 2: Ask Yourself, *"Why Do I Want This?"* This is probably the most important step in setting your goals, because it's what will give you the drive to achieve them. This step will help you to tap into your emotional state, allowing you to create change and the momentum you need to make your dreams become reality. Asking yourself the "why?" question will super-charge and magnetize your goals, so that you will be naturally drawn to take action towards their fulfillment. This second "why?" step ignites your desire, turbo-charges your energy level, and awakens your sleeping capabilities.

For example, why do you want to lose weight? Your answer needs to be a strong one if you're going to stick with it. Simply stating "to look good" is not enough. My reasons sprung from experiencing a traumatic miscarriage, and then giving birth to two healthy babies back to back. I was absolutely sick and tired of being overweight and out of shape, having to wear big black baggy clothes and big hair and tons of makeup to mask my heaviness. Also, I wanted to be healthy so I could have energy with my kids and be a better wife. These were super-strong reasons, which helped me to find my weight loss solutions and to stick with them. With that in mind, I urge to you take time on this step and to go deep within to find worthy reasons.

Step 3: Lastly, Ask Yourself, *"How Am I Going To Achieve My Goals?"* This part of goal setting gives you the necessary direction to take action. In order to think constructively about how you're going to reach your fitness goals, you have to break them down. You can't just say, "I want to lose some weight" or "I want to be healthier" or "I want to lose 30 pounds." These objectives are not specific enough to be goals. You must first have the ultimate vision of what you want, then be able to plan logically how to achieve it. Once you get specific, your goal doesn't seem so big and unattainable.

TIP #4: CHANGE YOUR RESULTS IN ADVANCE.

I love this Mind, Body and Soul principle. What does it mean, to change your results in advance? This means to have complete faith in the idea that you already have achieved what you have set out to accomplish. Now, you only have to take the necessary steps. This technique of knowing you can and will accomplish your goal is powerful because it takes the "I can't do it" part out from the start. You wipe out any and all self-doubt.

*"Everyone visualizes whether he knows it or not.
Visualizing is the great secret of success."*
—GENEVIEVE BEHREND

You must be able to visualize what it is you want to accomplish, in order for you to be off to an incredible start. Close your eyes and picture in your mind having already achieved your goals. See yourself celebrating your personal victory, what it feels like to actually accomplish what you set out to do, and how amazing it feels. Picture this image in high-definition color, not black and white.

Knowing vs. Hoping

When it comes to manifesting your dreams into reality, you must know that they will come true, rather than hoping they will. When working towards a desired outcome, you are more likely to make it come true when you know with conviction that you can and will make it happen. But if you simply hope for your goals to come true, it's not likely to happen. Tell yourself that you can, and you will. Don't focus on a weak wish or mere hope to achieve this. To hope is not strong enough. Knowing and believing with conviction is what will get you results. Attach strong emotion to how great you feel when you know that you can and will achieve your goals, and relish this memory.

MIND BODY AND SOUL DIET EXERCISE

Close your eyes and hope that your dreams and goals will come true.

How did that feel? Were the images in your mind clear and in color, or hazy and black and white?

Now close your eyes again, and visualize your goals, knowing with conviction that you can achieve them.

How did that feel? Did you see the images in your mind in color, or hazy in black and white?

For those of my clients with whom I have done this activity, I have seen that those who only hope, felt helpless, desperate, and out of control in making their dreams become a reality. Those who visualized with the conviction that they could and would make their dreams come true, saw their dreams and goals happening in crystal clear, high-def color.

Visualization

"Thoughts become things. Choose the good ones."

—MIKE DOOLEY, best selling author featured in *The Secret*

The power of visualization has been practiced for ages. It is the mental exercise where you picture yourself enjoying what you want. When you visualize, you create super-charged thoughts and feelings about living your dream life, the way you want it. You are setting yourself up for success by engaging your creative mind as your partner in seeing your life as you want it to be, inspiring you take the necessary actions to achieve it

I don't need to tell you that visualization is one of the most powerful mental exercises you can do. This is when it really helps to have a Mind, Body and Soul vision board, with actual pictures of your goals on it that you look at every day. Put your "before" picture up there to remind yourself why you're doing this, and also your "after" photo to draw you close to your goals.

How does it work and why? Thoughts, if powerful enough, are accepted by our subconscious mind as reality. Our mindset changes accordingly, along with our habits and actions, and this brings us into contact with new people, situations and circumstances.

Thought is the creative stuff that molds our lives, and attracts complementary stuff into our lives. If they are powerful enough, thoughts can travel from one mind to another, and be unconsciously picked up by others who are in a position to help us materialize our desires and goals.

Thought is energy, especially a concentrated thought laden with emotional energy. Thoughts change the balance of energy around us, and bring changes to the environment in accordance with them.

In my coaching sessions and consults I help many of my clients with the power of visualization. It helps them to overcome the limited thinking that boxes them in, not allowing them to grow upwards or to embrace new and positive changes in their lives. Visualizations helps to retrain the mind by opening it up to all powerful possibilities, both new and fresh. If you want to live a healthier, healed, happier life, visualize yourself doing so, knowing that it will come true, and materialize into reality.

TIP #5: FEED YOUR MIND.

Forget about diet soda and prepackaged, highly processed, so-called "health food" that you pick up at your neighborhood weight loss center or have sent to you through the mail. Start creating healthy meals with your own two hands. Enjoy the process of getting into your weight loss lifestyle mentally through becoming aware of what you do, what works for you, and what doesn't.

In Chapter 10, I've included my top favorite recipes for optimal mental and physical health. Our bodies and minds crave and need certain vitamins, minerals, and essential fatty acids. I will show you the essential nutrient-dense foods that are important because of the major roles they play in maintaining the excellent biological functioning of everything from your memory to your muscles. These include the super-foods I discuss in Chapter 9. Start with these recipes and branch out as you get comfortable cooking and trying new, fresh, healthy food. Remember, the fun of this new improved lifestyle is reawakening your dormant creative energy. You will fall in love with cooking again, and have so much fun creating super-healthy yet delicious meals that boost your mind, your body, and also feel good to your soul!

Mind Body and Soul Diet— Mental Health Top Ten

1. Tell yourself that you can, and you will. Remember Henry Ford's quote "Whether you think you can or you can't, you're right." It's true! We act and perform in accordance with our own beliefs. For example, if you think you can't, you won't even try. So believe that you can and you will!

2. End mental "civil war" by gaining clarity. Stop taking two steps forward, only to take two steps back. Like a gerbil on a wheel, you are going nowhere fast. So get clear on what you want, and go for it. Get out of your own way, and move towards your goal with conviction!

3. Let go of archaic, self-sabotaging belief systems. Old habits die slowly because they are driven by an outdated mindset. Replace your useless, sabotaging belief systems with new ones, in accord and in alignment with your new goals. Embrace new belief systems, which support your desired outcome.

4. Start using positive affirmations to make your mind your best friend, not your worst enemy: "I know I can do it," "There are people to help me along the way," "I can do anything that I put my mind to," and "I am not alone on my journey, as I can rely on my Higher Power to see me through."

5. Manifest your reality by choosing to know that you can do it, rather than hoping that you can. To manifest means to make

your thoughts materialize. We all manifest, so think positive thoughts all the time, and see the miracles happen in your life.

6. Don't ever let guilt shadow your success. Never allow anyone, including yourself, to guilt-trip you. Guilt is not a useful emotion.

7. Understand that there is no such thing as failure, only results. If we don't get the results we want, then this is the chance to try again with a different, new and improved approach. We can learn from our mistakes, and then reformulate our future attempts, getting better with every try.

8. Don't allow negative thoughts to rule in your head. Flip them around and completely reverse them until you get control of your mind. Tell yourself that your mind is your domain, and only allow self-loving, positive thoughts in.

9. Practice feeling gratitude, one of the strongest emotions, to ward off negativity and "joy-stealing." This is a great tool with which to prevent letting anyone steal your joy, even yourself. When you start to feel down or depressed, tell your mind and the universe that your joy is yours, and that no one will ever steal it or take it away. Tell yourself that you are too blessed to be stressed. It's a law of metaphysics that you can't be down or depressed when you are in a state of gratitude.

10. Don't allow anger and resentment to cloud your sunny future. "Let go and let God!" The Buddha stated, "Holding on to anger is like grasping a hot coal with the intent of throwing it at someone else; you are the only one who gets burned."

In order to help you to fully understand the power of your mind, let me offer this illustration. We all wake up with, say, $1,000 worth of mental space and mental energy to focus on our goals and to simply live our lives. If we spend $200 worth of our mental space and energy on thinking about a painful childhood memory, then we only have $800 left. If we then spend another $200 focusing on what our backstabbing ex-girlfriend did to us, then we only have $600 left. If we then spend another $200 on our cheating ex-boyfriend, and then another $200 on how horrible the office gossip queen is, then we only have a measly $200 worth of mental energy and focus to put towards our goals. So be ruthless in choosing what you focus on and what you think about. Be ruthless with your time, and make sure you use it wisely. Don't allow anybody or anything to steal your time away from you!

"Believe!" —JNL

Remember Vitamin C (confidence) and the F-word (faith)? I'd like you to add also Vitamin B: The Power of Believing! Most importantly, believing in yourself.

I started my own weight loss transformation when no one believed in me, when everyone around me judged me by my failed past attempts at losing weight. They doubted me; however, I believed in myself, and it worked! If you believe in yourself, it can work for you, too. You must have conviction that you will get healthy through the use of your mind. Believe that you can and you will.

CHAPTER 6

The Body

"The body doesn't lie.
It is your public billboard showing everyone whether
you are healthy or not." —JENNIFER NICOLE LEE

F rom Michelangelo's sculptures to the top fitness models in the industry, the power of the body is self-evident. The human body is one of the most studied, most celebrated and, sadly, also the most abused.

It's vital to treat your body with respect, to stop equating healthy living with just eating this food and doing that exercise. There's so much more to it. There are beauty rituals and exercises you can do every day, either at your local health spa or in the comfort of your own home, and on any budget, that will help you radiate beauty and health, to develop that glowing energy that money can't buy. The thing is, it doesn't really start until you embrace all of the success principles in *The Mind, Body & Soul Diet*.

I've been up and down on the scale more times than a kid goes up and down on a rollercoaster! I was finally able to "get off the merry go round" with Mind, Body and Soul Diet principles. I have been able to rev up my metabolism, start blasting fat faster, get lean quicker, look and feel younger, and build sleek and sexy feminine muscle tone, through the application of the philosophies and principles in this chapter.

I was once the "queen of cardio." I would walk into the gym so intimidated by all the different pieces of exercise equipment, not knowing what to do or how to use them. Also, I thought that the weight room was the "guys' side" of the gym, and it was safer for me to stick to the "women's side" with all the cardio machines. I knew I could get myself on a treadmill and press the start button and just walk. Doing cardio was easy, and I knew that at least I was doing something.

However, even though I lost weight with this strategy, I ultimately hurt my metabolism by not building strong muscle tone. It was the band-aid approach to quick weight loss, but my weight loss didn't last. I became a "skinny" fat person, by which I mean that, although I was thin, I still had more body fat than muscle tone. I was still flabby, with no energy.

I learned the hard way that it's not about the number on the scale, but about your energy level. It's not about being a certain dress size, but about having muscle tone to be stronger in your everyday tasks. It's not about being skinny, but about having more powerful endurance and stamina in life, to get more done. Yes, it's true that muscle weighs more than fat. So stop focusing on the scale, and instead, look at how you feel. Toning your muscles will help you rev up your metabolism, blast fat for good, increase your stamina, and give your body shape, structure, and definition. Keep in mind that a whole exercise program includes a balance of strength training, some cardio, and stretching for flexibility and de-stressing. Not only will you lose weight and gain muscle, but you will also help reverse many bio-marks of aging.

Whether you call it resistance training, weight training, or strength training, this is your body's Fountain of Youth. My personal experience, as well as numerous scientific studies, prove that going overboard on cardio can actually hinder you. What *will* help you is a balance between weight training and cardio, as well as incorporating relaxing exercises into your workout, such as yoga and Pilates. Even active meditation, teaching your body to be still and balanced in this chaotic, unbalanced world, is an exercise.

One of my clients, Sophia, consulted with me through ClubJNL. com. She confided in me, "JNL, I'm training for a marathon. I go to the gym and do spinning for an hour, and then I run on the treadmill for another hour, but I still don't look like you, strong with sleek and sexy feminine muscle tone." Her intentions were there, but having your intentions focused in the right direction is what will give you your desired results. She wanted the body of a sporty, athletic fitness model, but her focus was on the wrong kind of exercise. Again, our actions must be in alignment with our desired goals.

You're not going look like a fitness model no matter how much cardio you do, because fitness models don't do a lot of cardio. If you want to look like a fitness model, you must train like one. This involves training with weights and eating a healthy, balanced, high-protein, high-fiber, moderate carb diet. If your goal is not to be stick-skinny, but rather to be super-fit, with a feminine athletic build, then please see my FitnessModelProgram.com to get the program you should be following for a body that looks like it jumped right off of a top female fitness magazine cover.

Be methodical in your results. Intention is good, but it only gets you so far. Assess your situation and be flexible. Be adaptable. Ask yourself, "Is what I'm doing now giving me the results I want?" Use my goal-setting tips and ask yourself what you want, why you want it, and how you're going to achieve it.

At-Home Beauty Rituals

I've seen a lot of people lose weight only to look worse than what they did when they started. Even though they lost pounds, they also lost a lot of energy and vibrancy in their overall appearance. I have seen many who lost weight wind up with dry skin, dark circles under their eyes, whose faces take on a sunken-in appearance, with a shapeless, weak-looking physique. Believe me, abundant health is not only about losing weight; it's about looking your best, feeling your best, radiating health, and utilizing anti-aging beauty rituals. You can easily do this through some tried-and-true beauty and anti-aging rituals that I've discovered. The best part is that you will feel like absolute royalty after you get started incorporating them in your life—just the way you should feel!

Here are some great new habits that are easy to incorporate into your new healthy lifestyle.

Groom yourself for success. When you look good, you automatically radiate more confidence. Make a point to buy clothes that make you feel comfortable. Even though you may not be at your desired weight, its important for you to look and feel good—even if you aren't the size you want to be right now. If you don't know what looks good on you, go shopping with a trusted friend who has a sense of fashion, or buy a beauty magazine that offers tips on dressing for your body shape and size.

Enjoy a massage. We must realize that massage therapy is not a luxury, but an essential part of living a healed, whole, balanced lifestyle. One way I have found to get an affordable massage is by not relying solely on the high-end spas. If you go to your local massage therapy school, there are eager students ready to massage you at a discounted rate to get experience. Seek those students out and even have them come to your house. I have a massage table in my home so I can enjoy massages much more frequently without spa prices.

Create a spa environment in your home. I drink hot tea religiously, because of its antioxidant effects. One inexpensive spa treatment you can do at home is an Epsom salts bath. You can buy Epsom salts at your local pharmacy for a few dollars. Add it to a hot bath to mineralize your body and help draw out the lactic acid built up from working out. It also de-stresses and relaxes you.

Enjoy a glass of red wine. Believe it or not, red wine has been scientifically proven to dramatically decrease the number-one killer among women, heart disease, by a whopping 33 percent. It's also rich in antioxidants, so cheers to your health!

Have a chunk of extra-dark chocolate. This is why I love the Mind, Body and Soul Diet. The antioxidants in a chunk of extra-dark chocolate (85 percent cocoa) will actually help you fight off cancer-causing free radicals and boost serotonin levels in your mind, so you feel better and have a better outlook on life.

Indulge in super berries. These, too, are full of antioxidants, those cancer-fighting free radicals. They're also great for your hair, skin, and nails. Enjoying blueberries, raspberries, or strawberries dipped in dark chocolate with a glass of red wine is a beauty ritual I perform weekly. Every Friday after a long workweek, I have a hot bath with a glass of red wine with dark chocolate and my super berries. What a super fit, yet super yummy and indulgent way to start the weekend! And it's not even expensive.

Drink green tea. While doing research for this book in China, where longevity is common, I saw firsthand the enormous consumption of all sorts of tea and the effects it had on its consumers. Green tea's benefits are astounding.

Stimulate all your senses. Infuse your room with mood-enhancing aromatherapy oils and scents. Dim the lights and light a scented candle. After your hot bath, enjoy lounging on your bed in your most plush robe. Massage your feet with healing oils and then put on your softest socks. Treat yourself like the queen that you are!

Make your home your sanctuary. Your home is your solace away from the noisy world. It's your sacred space that is filled with love, friendship, and relaxation. See your home not as a bunch of walls with a roof on it, but rather as a shrine of health. Replace the candy bowl with a fresh fruit bowl. Have a special place for your workout area. Create a small meditation area. And always keep it clean, as cleanliness is next to Godliness! The more relaxing, peaceful, and healthy your home is, the fitter you will become, too.

Use supplements for beauty, energy, and anti-aging benefits. Nutritional supplements can actually help you to look and feel younger, and also may prevent many age-related illnesses. Vitamins, essential fatty acids (EFA's), joint nutrients, memory nutrients, nutrients for energy, antioxidants, and nutrients that boost immunity are all essential to obtain and maintain optimal health. Take your daily supplements as a beauty, energy, memory, and anti-aging ritual, knowing that they will increase your mental and physical capacity while also reversing your biological age.

Detox in your tub. Soaking in red desert clay is an inexpensive yet excellent way to detox the entire body. Red desert clay has a remarkable drawing effect, with the power to pull positively charged toxins out of the body, safely and effectively through the pores of the skin. It has the strongest ionic charge (pulling power) available. Toxins stick to the clay particles to assist in removing them.

Aromatherapy—Arouse Your Senses with The Power of Scents.
Of all our senses, our ability to smell is one of the most powerful. In fact, scents were considered so important in the beauty rituals of ancient Egypt that a nose hieroglyph was used in every word that meant "pleasure" or to be "pleased." Today we call this practice of using volatile plain oils, including essential oils, for psychological and physical well being, aromatherapy.

In aromatherapy, there are many scents with which to combat negative emotions or conditions, and to evoke positive ones. For instance, if you are struggling with anxiety, you can use cedarwood or rose scents. And if you want to gain confidence, you can use jasmine, rosemary, or grapefruit. To evoke feelings of peace and tranquility you can use bergamot, ylang ylang, sandalwood, or geranium.

Facials at Home: Facials are some of the most popular spa treatments. Professional facials can help maintain the elasticity and tone of your skin for a longer time. But they can be very expensive and time-consuming. I've created some great at-home recipes for when you are short on time and your budget needs a break.

1. *Salt Glow*: A very popular spa treatment that helps to eliminate dead cells, and makes your skin soft and radiant. Take ½ cup of sea salt and mix with ½ cup of cold pressed almond or apricot oil. Apply gently to wet skin. Rinse and moisturize.

2. *Caribbean Salt Glow:* Mix ½ cup of sea salt with ½ cup of cold pressed almond or apricot oil, 1 Tbsp of lime juice, and 2 tablespoon of coconut oil for extra moisture and to add a relaxing tropical scent. Apply gently to wet skin. Rinse and moisturize.

3. *Banana-Avocado Mask:* This recipe will nourish your skin. You will need ½ of an overripe banana, ½ of an overripe avocado, 2 Tbsp plain full-fat yogurt, and 1 tsp olive oil. Mash all ingredients together, mixing well. Apply liberally to face and neck. Place cool cucumber slices on your eyes. Leave on 20-30 minutes, then rinse with warm water.

4. *Tomato-Lemon Mask:* This will gently exfoliate. You will need 1 overripe tomato, 1 tsp fresh-squeezed lemon juice, 1 tsp instant oatmeal. Blend until smooth. Apply to face, place cucumber slices on your eyes, let soak 20 minutes, rinse with warm water and moisturize.

5. *Peach Mask:* This will tighten and tone your face, leaving it feeling youthful and taut again. You will need 1 ripe peach, 1 egg white, 1 tsp plain full-fat yogurt. Peel and pit peach. Blend together with egg white and yogurt till smooth. Pat gently onto face, place cucumber slices on your eyes. Leave on 20-30 minutes. Rinse with cool water.

6. *Honey-Almond Mask:* You will need 1 Tbsp honey, 1 egg yolk, ½ tsp almond oil, and 1 Tbsp yogurt. Mix all together, apply later to face, place cucumber slices on your eyes. Leave on 20-30 minutes. Rinse with warm water and moisturize.

Full Body Exfoliation: Your skin is the largest organ. We must exfoliate it weekly, helping it to shed dead skin cells, and revealing fresh, new, younger skin. Daily moisturizing is also essential to maintain the skin's overall health and elasticity. Here are some of my favorite full-body exfoliation recipes.

1. *Brown Sugar Scrub:* You will be glowing and feeling super sweet after one of my super Brown Sugar Scrubs. You will need ½ cup of brown sugar, 2 heaping Tbsp of almond oil, plus 3 to 5 drops of your favorite essential oil. Mix well and apply to wet skin, massaging gently. Rinse with warm water and apply your favorite moisturizer.

2. *Pina Colada Bath Scrub:* This is a bath that is both moisturizing and exfoliating. It uses the same ingredients as the famous cocktail. So enjoy soaking in a full body "cocktail" that will leave you feeling relaxed and refreshed! You will need 2 cups of pineapple juice, 1 cup coconut milk, 1 cup of milk, and 1 cup of powdered milk. Mix in blender, pour into your warm bath water, and soak for 10-15 minutes while sipping on some cold lemon or lime water. Close your eyes and feel the Caribbean sea breeze!

3. *Strawberry Lemon Drop Scrub:* Both sweet and tangy, this scrub will leave you feeling reenergized and super soft! You will need the grated zest of one lemon, ½ cup of sugar, ½ cup of sea salt, ½ cup of crushed strawberries, and 1 cup of sweet almond oil or olive oil. Mix all ingredients together and apply to wet skin, in a gentle circular motion. Shower off with warm water.

As you can see, at-home spa treatments can be both fun and inexpensive. So have fun with these recipes and rituals! For more great at-home beauty and spa treatments, please visit www.MindBodyandSoulDiet.com.

Mind, Body and Soul Diet Tools, Tips, and Techniques

TIP #1: STOP FAILING TO PREPARE.

Procrastination is the number one thing that unsuccessful people do. I love the saying "If you fail to prepare, then prepare to fail." Another nugget of truth is, "Plan your work and then work your plan." In order for you start "training" yourself to take positive action and steps towards creating your success, use the pleasure vs. pain technique. Push yourself towards your goals by linking immense pain to waiting until the last minute and not preparing yourself for success. And then pull yourself closer to your desired achievements by linking great amounts of pleasure to taking positive action and steps towards your goals.

Elizabeth, one of my clients, could never seem to make it to a workout. I asked her if she set out her workout clothes the night before, or if she had preplanned her workout schedule for the week, or if she had even packed her gym bag. She said no, she was not taking any of these three action steps. No wonder she could never find the time to exercise. She didn't prepare, and she didn't treat herself or her workouts with the respect they deserved.

Start treating your workouts like they were important business meetings that you cannot be late to, call in sick to, or just not show up for, with the most important person in the world: you. There are many ways to "fool" yourself into working out, because sometimes we need to just get up and moving onto our "upward spiral." I call it "setting yourself up for success." One way to ensure you won't bail on your workouts is to prepay for a bulk number of training sessions or classes in advance, so you know that if you miss one you've lost the money.

Often, hiring a personal trainer or having an exercise buddy will keep you on track. Always have a pre-packed gym bag in your car or at your office. One the same note, plan your meals for the week so you won't end up eating accidently or finding yourself at a vending machine or fast food restaurant.

Tips on how to never skip a workout again:

- Watch your favorite TV show while you are working out. Schedule your workout during your favorite TV show!

- Read a fitness magazine on your elliptical. Use the power of visualization; you are what you see! In the magazines, you will see lots of other people working out, which will motivate you and keep you moving. And if you need to get your little fix of "celebrity gossip," make it a point to buy one of the celebrity weekly magazines, but only allow yourself to read it during your cardio workout session. This little trick will work into anchoring you to your workout— even if you need to bribe yourself a little bit with an indulgence like reading all of the latest celebrity fashion do's and don'ts and Hollywood gossip.

- If you get bored easily, download new songs or even TV shows onto your ipod. This will keep you moving and grooving. Music has an amazing power. Download all of those favorite tunes that always make you want to get up and dance. These "power playlists" will keep you motivated and energized. Now remember, the faster and more upbeat the songs are, the more likely you will be to work out longer and harder. And put your songs on shuffle, so your curiosity will be stimulated to hear what song will randomly play next. It's like having the best of both worlds; you know you will love the next song because you downloaded it, but you won't know exactly which song it will be.

• If you are like me, you hate letting people down and cancelling plans. Pick at least one time a week for you and a close friend to be workout buddies together. This way, you won't let them down by not showing up, and you won't show up late. You will have a lot more fun and be a lot less likely to skip out. If you are competitive like me, you will want to keep up with your friend, or even push yourself a little bit harder.

• Try out a new gym class. Most gyms offer a variety of exercise classes, and this is your opportunity to be physically stimulated in new and different ways. Keeping you and your body guessing will also banish the boredom. Think of it this way; you already paid for the gym membership, so you may as well get your money's worth.

If you prepare, you will not give yourself the excuse to procrastinate. Lay out your workout clothes the night before, so that when you wake up, you have your clothes ready. Put a gym bag in your car, so that after or before work you can go straight to the gym to exercise. And on those super hectic busy days, where you can't get to the gym, set up a small home gym with some dumbbells, a mat, a stability ball, and a bench. This at-home gym set-up is great, too, for when you want to work out first thing in the morning. All you have to do is wake up, brush your teeth, and bang out your workout right at home. You might consider investing in a great piece of exercise equipment, in case it's raining and you don't feel like going to the gym. You can also purchase exercise DVDs. You pop one in, press "play," and work out. It's that simple.

In conclusion, stop making excuses and stop sabotaging yourself! Set yourself up for success. That's how you can start treating your workouts and yourself with the respect deserved.

TIP #2: USE THE "OUT OF SIGHT, OUT OF MIND/IN SIGHT, IN MIND" PRINCIPLE.

To prevent accidental eating, don't keep trigger foods that you know you've got a weakness for around you. Don't even bring them into the house. Just like the Good Book says, sometimes temptation is so powerful that you have to actually physically remove yourself from it in order to be safe. Don't set yourself up for failure by allowing your favorite cheat foods in your home and kitchen.

One of my coaching clients, Susan, told me that she used this success principle at her kids' birthday parties. She has always had a struggle with one of her most favorite foods—cake! She's a mom to five kids, all under the age of 10, so that means a lot of birthday parties. At least once a month she has to either throw a birthday party for one of her kids, or attend her kids' friends' parties. Every time she goes to a birthday party, she has to physically remove herself from the buffet table and the cake. She also makes it a point to eat before the parties, setting herself up for success by utilizing the power of anticipation. She anticipates that there will, of course, be cake and other unhealthy food options at the party, so she always has a pre-party meal.

Another coaching client, Stephanie, told me that she used to have a candy jar in her house. She was raised with a candy jar in her home as a little girl, and naturally she thought that it was something that every home had. But using the out of sight, out of mind/in sight, in mind principle, she has since replaced the sugary temptations with a fruit bowl and a nut jar. The candy is out of her sight, so it's out of her mind. She's set herself up for success by replacing the unhealthy trigger foods with the healthy ones. Now she sees the healthy food options, is naturally drawn to them, and enjoys them.

> **MBS DIET FIT TIP:** Always make sure that you're eating every two to three hours. Remember: Eat breakfast like a queen, lunch like a princess, and dinner like a pauper. Breakfast is the most important meal of the day because it works with your metabolism, revving it up for the rest of the day.

Stephanie also sets herself up for success by getting easy-to-eat, highly portable healthy snack options, such as precut vegetables with hummus, reduced fat string cheese, and fruits that she can grab with a handful of nuts.

TIP #3: PLAN YOUR SUCCESSES AND BUDGET YOUR TIME WISELY.

Successful people are always planning their success and using their time wisely. We all have the same amount of time, 24 hours a day. However, unsuccessful people and successful people utilize their time very differently. Hurried, frazzled, and frustrated people wait until the last minute and don't look at life like a chess game, always seeing things five steps ahead. Successful, relaxed, and centered people plan, plan, and then plan some more! Mastermind your own weight loss success by planning your workouts, grocery shopping, and meal preparation time into your calendar and schedule. You must become relentless in properly managing time, placing your family and your priorities first, and learning to ignore other's demands and distractions.

I coach my fitness clients to pick out one day to do their grocery shopping and schedule it into their day planners like an appointment.

This planning activity will ensure that they buy healthy groceries for the entire week, instead of rushing to the grocery store at the last minute when they're hungry, only to impulsively buy unhealthy foods.

In addition, pre-plan your workouts at the start of the week. I use Sunday as my workout-planning day. Knowing exactly what days I will train, what body parts I'll be concentrating on, and what classes I will take helps me to get clear on my goals and to stay focused. Planning ahead takes the confusion out of your week, and you then can budget your other important activities around your workout times.

Also, plan when you will prepare meals. You may find cooking several things at the beginning of the week and freezing them for quick meals later in the week works for you. You may want to cook a bit extra so you have leftovers for lunch the next day. Whatever you do, make sure you are scheduling time to make healthy meals for yourself. Again, I use the quiet time I have on Sunday to prepare and plan out my meals for the week. I love to start off my week on a positive note, with my grocery shopping done, my workouts planned out, and my cooking and food preparation done as well. You too will see that your weeks just flow better, you are less frazzled come Friday, and you're still on your super healthy fitness high. Make your time work for you, instead of you working for your time!

> MBS DIET FIT TIP: I usually do my grocery shopping early on Sunday morning, to save time when the store is the least busy, so I can get in and get out quickly, thus again saving time—a trick of the super successful. Try to pick a day and time when the grocery store is less crowded to use your time more efficiently.

TIP #4: DON'T OVERTRAIN.

Overtraining can do more damage to your mind, body and soul than good. Overtraining can actually create stress in the body, causing you to become unbalanced and leading you to gain weight. If you're training like a football player, you're going to start eating like a football player—and then start looking like one! In addition to weight gain, overtrainging can make you more susceptible to injuries and chronic fatigue, and can even cause your menstrual cycle to stop. Remember that you don't have to hurry or do more to lose weight. When you exercise and eat right, it will happen naturally.

Forty-five minutes of weight training with fifteen to twenty minutes of cardio afterward each day is all you need. Schedule weight training two days on, one day off.

Below is a sample week taken from my Fitness Model Program at www.FitnessModelProgram.com.

- Monday: Forty-five minutes upper body weight training, followed by fifteen to twenty minutes of low-impact cardio.

- Tuesday: Forty-five minutes of lower body weight training followed by fifteen to twenty minutes of low-impact cardio.

- Wednesday: Fun cardio day! Train your abs for about thirty minutes and then follow with thirty minutes of a favorite cardio of your choice. Pick a dance class at your gym, pop in that new workout DVD, or get outside and enjoy exercising outdoors.

- Thursday: Forty-five minutes upper body weight training, followed by fifteen to twenty minutes of low-impact cardio.

- Friday: Forty-five minutes of lower body weight training followed by fifteen to twenty minutes of low-impact cardio.

- Saturday: Same as Wednesday. Thirty minutes of abs training plus thirty minutes of a fun low-impact cardio of your choice.

- Sunday: Active rest day. Take the day off, and plan in a cheat meal if you want. In order to keep yourself on track, do your grocery shopping, plan your workouts, and then also plan and prepare your meals for the week.

For a more complete workout guide, please visit www.FitnessModelProgram.com

Top Ten Directives for Optimal Physical Health

1. Educate yourself about weight training. Most gyms offer one to two free sessions with a personal trainer that will help you get comfortable with lifting weights. Don't let working out "on the guy side of the room" intimidate you. Weight training is a stream of the Fountain of Youth, and you deserve to enjoy its benefits.

2. Don't worry about "bulking up." I have learned that women actually need to lift a little heavy weight in order to build the right amount of muscle tone. You're not going to get huge; you'll actually be whittling down and becoming tighter, smaller in size, and more compact.

3. Pencil in your workouts as important business meetings with the most important person in the world; you! Aim not to be late, cancel, or call in sick to these important meetings with yourself. This time is a gift to you.

4. Remember that your body is a temple. Engage in energy-increasing exercises and beauty rituals to show it respect and love.

5. If you don't know where to start, hire an expert. Find someone that has achieved the results you want, and watch how they're training and eating. If you desire a more intense, one-on-one private consultation with me, you may apply for a consultation at www.ClubJNL.com

6. Work out smarter, not harder. There is such a thing as overtraining. Follow my FitnessModelProgram.com, or www.GetFitNowWithJNL.com to see the exact workouts that I do, the foods that I eat, and the supplements that I use to get an award-winning, show-stopping physique.

7. Enjoy being creative! Ask yourself, "What are my favorite meals? How can I tweak these recipes to make them healthy?" If you love Italian food, look at your favorite Italian recipes and become your own concoction queen: see how you can remake your old favorites into lower-fat, lower-carb versions. If you need more recipes, log onto www.GetFitNowWithJNL.com and you will see many of my "JNL-approved" recipes!

    Don't only be creative with your meals, but with your physical activity as well. Who said that getting in shape equaled getting on top of a big machine and pressing the "start" button? Ask yourself, "What are the exercises I love to do most?" or "What sport have I always wanted to try, or to get better at?" For instance, if you love to play tennis, join a tennis club. You can also hire an instructor who will help you strengthen your backhand or give you a better edge on your game. If you never have done a spinning class, but always wanted to try one, then enroll in the next class.

8. Set yourself up for success. Set your gym clothes out the night before. Create a small home gym. Buy exercise DVDs. Keep a gym bag in the car, and at work.

9. Don't set yourself up for failure by allowing your favorite fat-gaining trigger foods where you'll be tempted by them. Instead, place quick, portable, grab-and-go healthy food options around you, and surround yourself with people with similar healthy lifestyle goals and habits. If you are at parties where you know your favorite unhealthy trigger foods will be, have a pre-party meal to fill you up and take the edge off of your hunger.

10. Get a handle on stress with mind/body exercises such as active meditation, yoga, and Pilates. These de-stressing exercises will help you gain balance in an unbalanced world, so that you are not gaining weight or aging more quickly due to stress.

Start your complete transformational program with self-love and self-respect. You have the power to make it creative and fun. Enjoy your fitness freedom by growing upwards from the outdated belief system that being in shape is limited to the boring calorie-in/calorie-out mentality, and open your mind to trying new and different tools. Once you see that you are more powerful than you ever thought you were, you will have multitude of useful tips, tools, and techniques at your fingertips, to use in fighting and winning the war on fat. Rather than seeing being fit as torture or boring as you did in the past, you now are equipped and enlightened to make fitness fun, refreshing, and interesting. You will re-awaken your passion by being fit. You will fall in love with the new-found freedom that stems from living a fit lifestyle. There will never be a dull moment in your new, healthy life, which you'll live full of self-love and self-respect.

An important key to long-term fitness success is to choose to enjoy the process of being fit. You noticed how I said "choose," because we do have a choice. We have the power to see fitness as torturous, or as fun and enjoyable. This key to fitness success, choosing to view living a healthy lifestyle as fun, is crucial. If you link pleasure to your new-found freedom in your life, you will stick with it. Remember how we've all had those great New Year's resolutions, but only stuck with them for a couple of weeks? Have you really wondered why your past attempts at developing new, healthy habits lasted such a short time? It's because you didn't view being fit, or working out, or eating healthy, as fun! This time around, it's different for you, and yes—the past does not equal the future. So cheers to you for finally getting it right, and congratulations on making fitness fun and a new part of your life.

Mind, Body and Soul Diet Online Community

If you need inspiration, make sure you visit www.MindBodyAndSoulDiet.com There you will find an online community of other Mind, Body and Soul Diet fitness friends, a variety of exercises, workouts, de-stressing practices, and beauty ritual ideas. I warmly invite you to log on, to create new fitness friendships, network, and enjoy researching new fun ways to make your life healthier, healed, and happier!

CHAPTER 7

The Soul

"You are never alone, no matter how lonely, desperate, or lost you may feel. You don't have to go through your life's journey all by yourself. You will always have your Higher Power guiding you and helping you, which you may lean on for strength to carry you through. " —JNL

"Spirituality is a domain of awareness."
—DEEPAK CHOPRA

No matter what our spiritual beliefs, most of us acknowledge that there is something greater than we are, some force behind this immense, immeasurable universe and our existence. We are the creation of something greater than we can imagine. Our minds, bodies, and souls are masterpieces, wonderful works of endless detail. In this chapter, I'm going to discuss the power of the soul with a powerful intention in mind; to reawaken that spiritual energy within you. Even when you feel lonely, depressed, or down and out, you will always have your Higher Power to lean on. It will guide you out of your downward spiral, and onto your upward spiral of success.

I want to use the analogy of a glove to help you understand this concept. If you place a glove on a table, it's just going to lay there, motionless. Think of that glove as your body. Now, when you put your hand inside the glove and start wiggling your fingers, the glove begins to move. Think of this as your spirit, making your body move. When our bodies have been laid to rest and our physical beings becomes ashes and dust, our souls live on.

Thus, even when your body is weak, your soul can still be strong. In your darkest, loneliest hour when you feel as though you can't go on anymore, you must rely on your soul's strength to kick in. This is the point at which you can turn bitter, allowing life to get the best of you, or you can become better, growing stronger through your life's challenges.

If you think that your spiritual side is weak, think again. You are spiritually stronger than you even realize. It's my joyous passion as a life coach to help you to recognize that you are indeed connected to the universe and, through that realization, to help you to work at achieving your true potential. As a life coach, it's my duty to be an objective person, helping you to see the things that you don't notice. I am here to help you achieve your utmost potential. And in order for you to really take the brakes off of your success, you must reconnect with your spiritual side.

If you think that you are not spiritual, think again. In all reality, your life is your biggest school of spirituality. Think briefly over your

> **MBS DIET FIT TIP:** Make living a fit lifestyle fun, creative and interesting! This is a big success key to insuring your life long fitness success. For instance, become a Concoction Queen! Learn how to create low fat, high fiber nutrient dense meals, which mimic your favorites. Take your favorite meals, and tweak the recipes, thus allowing you to prepare them without all the unnecessary fat, salt, sugar, and carbs, to revamp them into a healthier version.

life up until this point. Look at all of your past mistakes, failures, and successes. These special experiences, good and bad, have all served you as spiritual exercises, building your spirit's strength. I know first hand and with deep conviction that I could not have achieved any of my successes without relying on my Higher Power to see me through my everyday actions. My Higher Power helped me day in and day out to help me stick with it, and to never give up.

Here is a quick quiz to see if you are being spiritually enlightened, "spiritually fed" and inspired every day. Simply answer yes or no to all of the following questions. For every yes, give yourself a point.

Mind, Body and Soul Diet Spirituality Quiz

1. Do you daily praise yourself for your personal accomplishments?

2. Do you feel connected to your Higher Power, as if you are best friends?

3. Are you in tune with your sixth sense?

4. Do you daily rely on your Higher Power to make the right decisions, even when you are tempted to do otherwise?

5. Do you daily give thanks and praise for all of your blessings?

6. Do you keep irritation with life's little bumps in check, by looking at the larger picture?

7. Do you daily meditate for at least 5 minutes, write in your journal, or pray to give thanks?

8. Do you have spiritual mentors to whom you go for guidance or help, when you are struggling with issues?

9. Do you believe in miracles?

10. Do you believe that you attract what you truly want?

SCORE:

The more questions you answered "yes" to, the healthier you are, spiritually. If you answered "no" more often than "yes," you can benefit from some spiritual nourishment, and inspiration. Take another look at the questions to which you answered "no." These questions designate the areas you need to address to truly feel "alive" in your life, full of love, passion, and fulfillment. If you feel lonely, alone, and as if you are going through life all by yourself with no one to help you, then this chapter will help you to open your portal of spirituality, allowing you to enjoy true joy and happiness.

When we are suffering in many areas of our lives, it's a sign that we are living our lives in lack of spiritual enlightenment. This is not living a truly healthy life. If we are not daily being "spiritually fed," we are not living to our complete and full potential. And if we can lift up and re-shape up our bodies by working out, why can't we also aim to lift up and re-shape our spirituality? I want you to banish all negative past feelings towards being spiritual and spiritually connected. Being enlightened and knowing that your life is precious is a celebration. This chapter is devoted to you—a masterpiece in the making—who are in need of being energetically recharged, through being spiritually fed.

For instance, I have been in a so-called "happy" area in my life in terms of the material world, when I was at my desired weight. But I was suffering spiritually and I was not happy or fulfilled. I found it quite odd that I was thin, but not happy. I remember thinking to myself "I wanted to be this weight for so long, and I am finally here, but I am not happy. Why?" I only went on to gain all of the weight back. It was then that I understood the direct correlation between my health and permanent weight loss, and my spirituality. It was not until I made the effort to fill my spiritual void that I was able to outsmart life's most challenging moments and come out on top, healthy, healed, and happy. It was not until I started to "feed myself spiritually" that I was able to master lifelong weight loss, with no more yo-yoing up and down on the scale.

"Forgiving releases you from the punishment of a self-made prison where you are both the inmate and the jailer." —HOWARD MARTIN

FORGIVENESS

One way to heal yourself is through one of the most important Universal Laws; the law of forgiveness. The Good Book states "Forgive and you will be forgiven." Exercise this powerful principle by letting go of the past to embrace your beautiful future, free of bitterness and resentment.

This doesn't mean that what others have done to you isn't awful and unfair. Remember, holding onto resentment is like holding onto a hot coal. You're only burning yourself. If you're holding onto resentment and haven't forgiven those who have done wrong to you in the past, you're not freeing your life to create miracles and receive blessings that are yours for the taking. I urge you to forgive and forget. Here are some personal stories from some of my past clients, to help you liberate yourself also from your pain.

I coached Kathy, one of my clients, to use this powerful success principle of forgiveness. Her hurtful past memories had cannibalized her present state, and thus her future. Her husband had cheated on her, and it was eating her up inside, causing her to become bitter and angry most of the time. This pent-up anxiety, frustration, and hatred were spiraling out of control, causing her to emotionally eat. She had created "walls" around her emotions and her heart, but clearly she had to let go of the past so that she could move on and start enjoying life and other relationships again. I worked with her to release her anger and to forgive him, which allowed her to move onward and upward.

Another coaching client, Stella, had emotionally eaten most of her life. She had been badly abused growing up. To console herself through the pain she had suffered, she found comfort and even a kind of love through food. When I coached her to heal herself through forgiveness, she was able to get control of her emotional eating, and to start being healthier by exercising and eating optimally.

"Let go and Let God." —ANONYMOUS

Ultimately, as an expert who's listened to hundreds of consultations, I realize that one of the reasons that many of us find it impossible to forgive is this feeling of allowance. By this I mean that, when you consider forgiving another, you might feel as if you're granting that person permission to have committed his or her sin against you. Let me be clear; that isn't what you're doing by giving them your forgiveness. The power of forgiveness lies in the action of letting go. When you let go, you don't allow anybody or any past memory to further stain, taint, or haunt your present, thus stifling your future.

There is a powerful shift in energy when you forgive. You are starting the healing process. "Healing" is the most important word in this chapter. Healing will help you evolve from being a broken person, to putting your life back together again. Healing is the adhesive glue that can repair any broken soul.

"You must first want to be fit, and then do the exercises yourself. No one can exercise for you. The same is true of healing. You must want to be healed first, and then do the exercises to heal yourself." —JNL

No one can heal you, for you. You must do it yourself. Stop playing the victim and start being victorious! The amazing part is that we can heal ourselves, and we don't need to spend thousands of dollars on an expert to do so. It's this inner spiritual work that will actually liberate us in our own lives. It's about letting go of the negative past, and not allowing it to dwell in our present. Focusing on negative past events will put the brakes on your success and hold you back from progressing, not to mention draining you mentally, physically, and emotionally.

Remember: We all wake up with a $1000 worth of energy. If we spend $200 of that on what this person did to us in our childhood, and another $200 on what that person did to us five years ago, and another $200 on what that person said about us yesterday, and then another $200 on what this person is doing to us now, and finally another $100 of energy on how unfair life is, we'll have little to no energy to focus on our goals and spiritual growth! Stop wasting your energy playing the victim, and start healing yourself. Don't allow those negative experiences and less-than-worthy people to steal your present joy and future successes.

Forgiving someone is a powerful exercise. However, after you forgive them, this doesn't mean that you have to hang out with them, speak with them, or become friends again. The choice of whether or not to allow this person into your personal space again is entirely yours. The most important thing is to forgive them, so that the negative energy generated by your anger and pain won't continue to cloud your mind, force you to emotionally eat, or be drained physically.

Mind, Body, and Soul Tips, Tools, and Techniques

TIP #1: WRITE IT DOWN.

Write down all of the past wrongs that people have done to you on a piece of paper. Look at that piece of paper, and tell yourself and your Higher Power that you are healed and whole. Decide that you're letting go of the past, and that you will no longer allow your spiritual space to be taken up by these negative events. Then tear up that piece of paper and throw it away. Top performance coaches, award winning athletes and Olympic competitors all do this simple exercise, freeing up more mental and emotional space for their future achievements. It sounds like a simple exercise, but it's powerful and it works.

MBS DIET FIT TIP: Learning to "Let go and to let God" is an emotional and spiritual exercise that we must use many times in our lives. When a problem is bigger than us, and we can't solve it ourselves, learning to let go and let God is a sure way to help lessen the stress burden, thus not expending time and energy on things beyond our control.

TIP #2: JOURNAL EVERY DAY.

When you journal every day, not only do you get in touch with what's going on inside of you, but you can also track your successes. Journaling allows you to take an audit of your life so that you can embrace what is helping you, and let go of what is hindering you. It's also an excellent way for you to objectively see how you are spending your time, either in a positive way by exercising, or in a negative way by worrying or stewing over issues.

TIP #3: PRAY.

Prayer is one of the most powerful things you can do anywhere, at any time. There are many ways to pray. It can mean meditating in a quiet spot, closing your eyes while you lay peacefully on your couch or bed, or actually kneeling down with your hands held in the prayer position. The marvelous thing about prayer is the instant ability it gives you to call upon your Higher Power, wherever you are and whenever you need to. I personally use the power of prayer when I feel my body is weak, and I don't feel as if I have the energy to make it to my workout or go through my daily tasks. This activity of gratitude and reverence helps me to gets my body moving and my mind in a more productive place.

Prayer is a vital exercise for your spiritual growth. We exist to grow as spiritual beings, to learn from our past mistakes, and to find answers through relying upon our Higher Power. We can do that through active meditation, which is the power of prayer.

MBS DIET FIT TIP: Praying doesn't cost anything! It's a powerful activity which is free, can be done anywhere and at any time, and which yields amazing results. It helps you to get in tune so you may be that much more productive, centered, balanced and focused on what really matters. Plus your Higher Power is the best "expert" you can consult with and run to when you got a problem. Stop sharing your real problems with those who just may not understand or be able to help you, and go to your Higher Power.

TIP #4: FIND YOUR ALTER EGO.

Part of the spiritual journey is finding your alter ego. Everyone has an alter ego. Your alter ego is the stronger, hidden side to your personality. Connect with your alter ego, which is going to be your "very close friend" in helping you to become more successful and masterful in your life, and in achieving your goals. Many have even named their alter egos. My alter ego is La Tigra, which is Spanish for "tigress." It's that powerful female prowess that comes out to defend my honor if someone attacks it, to stand up for the things I believe in, and to protect my children.

The Alter Ego & Many Sides to a Woman's Soul

"In a single human being, there are many other beings, all with their own values, motives, devices. Some suggest we arrest these beings, force them into harness until they shuffle along like vanquished slaves. But to do this would halt the dance of wildish lights in a woman's eyes; it would halt her heat lightning and arrest all throwing of sparks." —CLARISSA PINKOLA ESTES, *Women Who Run With the Wolves*

Everyone has a fearless alter ego that comes alive during fight or flight. Getting in touch with your alter ego will be one of your most amazing experiences. Stand up for yourself when someone does you wrong. Be outspoken. Enjoy regaining your backbone and becoming vocal about what you want and what you deserve. It will help you to protect your goals, to become more confident in your abilities, and to fight for what you believe is right. Your life is wholly worthy of seeing your desires come true, and sometimes you need to rely upon your alter-ego to help you get that job done.

Many ask me, "Do I have an alter ego?" And the answer is a resounding "yes!" Everyone has an alter ego, just waiting to be awakened. If you don't think that you do, it's lying dormant inside of you. Use this book to help awaken the power inside you to help create the healthiest life that you deserve, a fit life that's worth fighting for.

TIP #5: PRACTICE RITUALS OF GRATITUDE.

"A Joyful Spirit is evidence of a grateful heart." —MAYA ANGELOU

The most important emotional state that is linked directly to spirituality is gratitude. When you're grateful for what you have, it's impossible to be negative, depressed, or fearful.

Practice rituals of gratitude daily. I begin and end my day with a special time in which I connect with my Higher Power and the universe. One of my favorite rituals is to recite my life's mission statement and mantras. Every morning I proudly recite mine. I then boldly share with the universe what I'm going to do today, asking for a guiding path to successfully get all that I need to do, done. I thank my Higher Power in advance for helping me achieve my tasks. Then, at the end of every day before I go to bed, I give thanks for all the small miracles that happened throughout my day, and for the energy and focus I had during the day to keep me on my upward spiral.

If you don't have your own life mission statement, now is the time to create one. You could use something like, "Thank you, Higher Power, for my strong, healthy, mind and body, and for my ability to work every day, to do good today, to make a positive difference today." Or "I thank you in advance for helping me become a better, fitter, more in-tune person every day. Please help me to be the best that I can be, no matter what is happening around me or in my life. Thank you for all of the miracles in my life." This is the fun part, where you get to create your very own life mission statement and mantras. Enjoy this time, because it's in the act of creating your mantras and mission that you grow the most, spiritually.

"Being grateful is like waking up. You must do it every day to feel totally alive and to have a successful day." —JNL

It's very difficult to maintain an attitude of gratitude in these challenging times. A powerful exercise in redirecting your focus is to zap all negativity right from the start. For instance, if you see or feel yourself getting negative, stop yourself, and start listing your blessings and what you are grateful for. This is a potent exercise to help get your mind and spirituality back on track, and moving in the right direction. Again, it's a law of metaphysics that you cannot be depressed or down when you are in a state of true gratitude.

"Most people are thinking about what they don't want, and they're wondering why it shows up over and over again." —JOHN ASSARAF, from *The Secret*

Think of your mind as a finely-tuned sports car. When you are being resentful and focusing on the bad things in your life, you are putting your gears into reverse, and keeping yourself behind in the race of life. When you are living a life full of joy, happiness, and gratitude, you are living it in 5th gear, racing towards your success, and enjoying every mile of the way. Aim at being grateful every day for all that you have, and you will see that more good things will be created in your life. Remember, you get more of what you focus on. So catch yourself when you are focusing on negative things, and redirect your focus by being grateful. Stop living in reverse, and start enjoying the ride of your life in 5th gear!

TIP #6: ALWAYS BLESS YOUR FOOD BEFORE YOU EAT IT.

One ritual of gratitude that I rarely see people perform anymore is the blessing of their food at meal times. Giving thanks over your meals is such an important exercise, no matter how simple or extravagant the meal. Make it a point to always give thanks for your nourishment, whether it's a simple peanut butter and jelly sandwich or a five-course supper at a lavish restaurant.

Why take the time to be thankful for your food? Well, for many reasons. Showing gratitude for your food shifts your energy into a super-charged, positive mode. It will put your mind into a zone of appreciation and you will instantly become more centered and balanced. Being at peace and relaxed while you eat will also help banish any emotional stress and deter overeating. Also, it will help you to eat healthier and to make better food choices. If you can banish any stress before eating, you are more likely to eat less and to enjoy eating healthier, energy-boosting foods.

Try this sample blessing: "Thank you for this nutritious meal. Thank you for blessing it so it may nourish my body and soul." This simple ritual of gratitude, right then and there, automatically transitions you to pay attention to what you're putting in your body and whether it is really healthy.

"I had these recipes that say do this, do that.
Who MAKES these rules?" — EMERIL LAGASSE

Cooking and preparing your own meals is, sadly enough, a rare activity for many individuals and families. The great thing about cooking is that it puts the passion back into creating healthy meals full of nutrients that are immense gifts to your body. Make it a goal to fall back in love with cooking. We all have a budding chef lying dormant inside of us, just waiting to be awakened. Preparing your family meals with your own two hands, with fresh herbs, intense spices, and unprocessed ingredients, benefits you in many ways. First of all, it heightens your awareness of what you are really putting into your body. Secondly, you can cut all of the unnecessary fat, calories, and sodium out of your meals. You are much more in control of what you are feeding your family and yourself.

"Cook when you are happy.
And be happy when you cook." — JNL

Your attitude while preparing your new healthy meals is also important when creating your recipes. Aim to be in a state of gratitude for all of the wonderful ingredients when you are cooking your meal. Be happy while you are in your kitchen—a place of celebration with friends and family.

Cooking for me is a type of therapy. I am able to unwind from my day, and get back to the important basics of life. Leave the stress at the kitchen doorway, and allow yourself to get fully immersed. Enjoy all the fresh wonderful smells, flavors, and seasonings while you cook and be grateful for them and this experience. You will be preparing your meals in a state of appreciation, and thus preparing them with love for yourself and your loved ones, which is beneficial to all.

When you sit down as a family, do not talk about any controversial or emotionally-charged topics. Leave those for another time. Let's get real here; there is enough stress out there in the real working world. And we all know it's stress that causes us to emotionally eat, sabotaging our healthy weight loss efforts. When you come home, make it a point to only speak about the nice things that happened to you during the day, even if you really have to dig for something to say. Don't start any conversation that will lead to heated debates. Instead, choose to engage in conversion that brightens up everyone's mood.

Top Ten Directives for Spiritual Health

1. Rely on your Higher Power. It's stronger than you will ever be. You don't have to lose weight and get healthy alone. When the process is challenging, your Higher Power will see you through and help you to continue.

2. Find a community. Call upon an expert to help guide you and give you the success principles that are going to help you. You can consult with me one-on-one by applying for a consultation at www.ClubJNL.com. I'm always just an e-mail away. Just fill out the application and I'm there to listen to your problems and help you find the answers.

3. Share and connect with yourself. Even if no one is there to listen, write about how you're feeling in your journal.

4. Don't be afraid to vent. There's great relief in venting your frustrations, so don't feel as if you have to keep them bottled up inside. Remember to nurture your alter-ego and to use this spiritual energy in a positive way.

5. View learning as a never-ending process. If you feel like there's nothing else to learn, you might as well put yourself in the grave because life will no longer be passionate, fun, or interesting. A key to having vitality, zest for life, and keeping yourself young at heart is to ask yourself what you can learn today and how it can spiritually enlighten and empower you. Become engaged with other people who are on a similar journey, and learn from their past failures and their current successes.

6. Detox your soul. We've been so brainwashed and browbeaten by our surroundings and society into fitting into these little boxes that we just don't know where to start anymore. I want you to detox your mind and your spirituality. Banish the self-limiting beliefs that keep you trapped from growing mentally, physically, emotionally, and spiritually.

7. Be optimistic. Especially in today's world of upheaval and uncertainty, being optimistic is important. It will help to rebalance you in this unbalanced world. Being positive keeps you centered and focused. People create drama in their lives all the time by engaging in gossip and other negativity; why not create spiritual miracles, joy, peace, happiness, prosperity, and love instead? Use optimism in

a realistic way by making a plan of action and following through.

8. Visualize yourself as successful already. This is a spiritual exercise that is essential to the soul diet. Feed yourself spiritually by using the power of visualization and seeing yourself living the life you want to live and having that healthy dream body you want.

9. Have a strong will. When the world comes at you from all angles, when nothing is going your way, the winner is the one who picks herself up just one more time. Remember, it's not about being perfect; it's about being persistent.

10. Connect with your Higher Power on a daily basis through the power of prayer and positive affirmations. Start your day off by stating aloud, "Thank you for my strong, healthy mind and body and for the ability to create the life of my dreams." End your day every day by thanking your Higher Power again for the energy to get things done and stay on your upward spiral.

IS YOUR SOUL A DRY DESERT FILLED WITH BITTERNESS, OR A ROBUST, VIBRANT RAIN FOREST FILLED WITH LOVING ENERGY?

Your soul, just like your body and your mind, expands and grows. It has an identity. If it's bitter, dry, and jaded, how can a seed of optimism and prosperity grow? Your soul needs to be open to positivity. If you feel little or no compassion, or if life has taken the joy out of you, and made you jaded, then use inspiring mission statements and mantras to help reawaken your spirit. This simple activity is powerful, and will help you embrace a newer, healthier lifestyle.

So, if you feel like your soul is sour because of past resentments you've built up over the years, remember the power of forgiveness, of positive affirmations, of looking at the happiest times in your life, and understand that your joy is yours to enjoy. Don't allow anybody or anything, not even yourself, to steal your own joy! Then your soul will become that rich, fertile soil that will reap a beautiful harvest, a landscape of rolling hills and boundless abundance. Your heart and your soul will be unhardened and become fertile ground again, from which many seeds of prosperity, abundance and joy can grow.

Let's Talk About Sex, Baby!

"Despite what you may have been conditioned to believe, sexual desire is sacred and virtuous."
—DEEPAK CHOPRA from *Grow Younger, Live Longer*

Part of our spiritual energy is our sexual energy. In today's society, we are misled to believe that the act of loving someone is merely a physical and carnal exercise. However, the root of all love is from the spirit and our souls. If our soul and spirit are not engaged in our sexual energy, then it's only an act of the body and flesh, with no real loving emotions attached. This is where the line is drawn; if no love is involved, a sexual act is more of domination and control over another person's dominion or body. It's animalistic in nature, and not blessed with the greatest gifts of all, which are the gifts of love and light.

Answer this question: Have you ever had a sexual experience that left you feeling empty, lonely, used, and sad afterwards? These feelings are signs telling you that this sexual act derived from the desires of the body, not the love from someone else's spirit. If you ever truly enjoyed a sensual experience, and afterwards felt loved, secure, respected and admired, those feeling are telling you that the sexual act stemmed from a deeper love, from one's soul.

I am saddened as a life coach to hear in my numerous consultations how poorly satisfied many of my clients are in their own sex lives. Suffering from little to no libido, not remembering the last time they felt attractive or aroused, and also suffering from the poor quality of the intimate experience with their loved one, are just a few of the many examples that I have heard. Knowing this, I knew that this section of the soul chapter must address the importance of enjoying our sensual energy, as our creative sexual energy is an extremely important part of our spiritual side.

It's as simple as this—you can increase the quality of your life by nurturing your true sensual energy. The benefits of a healthy loving sex life are immense. Here is a quick list of the advantages to creating a healthy sex life:

- Reduction in stress.
- Boosts the immune system.
- Live a longer and more enjoyable life.
- Sex strengthens pelvic floor muscles.
- Burns calories, a healthy form of cardio.
- Increase in cardiovascular health by reducing the chances of a fatal heart attack.
- Boosts positive self esteem.
- Sex improves intimacy. Having sex and orgasms increases levels of the hormone oxytocin, the so-called love hormone, which helps us bond and build trust.

Not only does having a healthy sex life increase the quality of your life, there is a flip side. Exercising will also increase the quality of your sex life. They go hand in hand. If you exercise, you will have more flexibility, stronger muscle tone, and more sexual confidence. Exercising to increase sexual pleasure is especially important for moms. Women who have gained weight while pregnant have had their abdomen and pelvic area stretched out and weakened during pregnancy and childbirth. Exercising will help tighten and tone up the mid-section and lower pelvic area, allowing them to enjoy sex much more.

"What is love?
Love is the soul in motion." —ANONYMOUS

Sexual energy is the innate, creative, loving energy of the universe, yet it is not limited simply to having sex. Think about the last time you really felt alive, vibrating on every level in this existence. Was it when you were looking out from an oceanfront balcony, watching the sunset? Or stargazing on a clear, quiet night? Or the first time you saw your newborn baby? Being passionately aroused in your spirit and then allowing your physical body to feel the vibration of this, is also a sensual experience. Your hair might seem to grow on your head; you may get goose bumps, or the hair on the back of your neck may "stand up." These are physical signs of your soul being aroused.

I urge you to also break away from the archaic notion that to "make love" means only the contact of genitals. You can "make love" daily with your loved one in so many other ways. A strong kiss, a tight squeeze, a sincere glance into your lover's eyes, a phone call, or a gentle touch will express your true feelings of love, and transmit sensual energy their way.

Did you know that the skin is the body's largest organ? On the average adult it covers about 3,000 square inches, receives about 1/3 of the blood circulating in your body, and has hundreds of thousands of nerve endings that produce sensation. I like to remind my clients that a simple touch of pure love to your partner's hand, arm, leg, shoulders, or any other contact with their skin can also be intimate. Enjoy your partner's body, all of it, not just those certain areas which we are led to believe are the only targets for sexual arousal. The entire body, top to bottom, and the mental and spiritual components, are all portals of love.

Sexual exuberance and vitality is accessible to all. Nurturing and tending to your sensual energy is youth-boosting. This is why it's a gift. But, sadly enough, many abuse this gift of pleasure. The meaning that society has attached to the idea of having a healthy sex life has misled us. Extreme forms of unhealthy sexual expressions, such as pornography and casual group sex, have been so integrated into our mainstream society that they seem almost normal. We must work as a community to return sacredness to the blessed act of intimacy. Treat your intimate relationship as a sacred act between you and your loved one, combining your two spirits into one.

How do we transform the typical everyday sex into an ethereal experience? We make the mental shift from "sex" to "holy ritual" where we take the time to prepare for our sacred act of sexual expression. I call it "setting the stage." Set the stage and create the arousing ambiance to your liking. It's much better to be intimate with your loved one while enjoying lit candles and soft music.

How to Set the Stage:

- Light candles
- Dim the lights
- Play soft music
- Scent the room with an appealing fragrance
- Give yourself the mental break from work mode, allowing yourself to be fully with your partner.
- Enjoy feeling as sexy and as womanly as possible, by celebrating your body by dressing yourself up in beautiful lingerie.
- Enjoy a warm bath before, or a shower with your partner.
- Massage each other gently, on the temples, head, neck and shoulders to help release any tension.

Your life's story will not be complete without a satisfying, loving, pleasing, and passionate love life. Your soul needs love to flourish and grow. If you feel that you are in a toxic relationship, one that is stifling and strangling your spirit, then make the bold step for the well-being of your soul to move on and allow yourself to heal. If you feel you can piece together this broken relationship to your mutual advantage, then seek counseling. I always believe that love is worth preserving and fighting for. If you are in a pleasing relationship and your partner is open to explore the glorious realm of passion with you, then embrace this special opportunity, allowing both of your souls to be bound as one through love.

For more information on how to strengthen your relationship with your Higher Power and to fortify your spiritual growth, please visit www.MindBodyandSoulDiet.com

Persistence Over Perfection

*"Being good consistently trumps being
perfect once."* —JENNIFER NICOLE LEE

P erfection does not exist in this reality. Therefore, do not set yourself up for failure by aiming to be perfect. I've always said that being good on a continual basis, trumps being perfect once. You're not ever going be perfect, even on your weight loss and self-improvement journey, so stop trying. Trying to be perfect will only frustrate you. Let go of that outdated belief system that perfection is obtainable. This all-or-nothing, black-or-white mindset doesn't serve you, it only holds you back. I have seen the scenario way too many times. You try to be perfect in your weight loss program, stressing yourself out, then letting yourself down. You then give up on yourself two weeks later.

Let's embrace the other side, which many of us rarely tap into, to really enjoy life and who we are. Think of being successful this way; you are perfect in your imperfections. You love yourself the way you are now, and you will only get better one day at a time. Having this kind of control will help you progress. Focus on being persistent to achieve a healthier lifestyle.

The Outer World and Our Inner World

Striving for perfection is a byproduct of our society—I call it the "outer world." We have no control over the outer world, but we do have control over our inner worlds.. I am speaking from my personal experience, as well as for many of my clients. You see, the only way we will truly achieve our goals is to focus on what we can control, and not waste time pleasing others or trying to control the outer world. To insure our success, we must shift our focus from the outside world which we can't control, to our inner world. We must focus on making sure we get to our workouts, eat optimally, and embrace this new, fresh outlook on life.

Clarity is Key

"Clarity is a key to success.
But being clear with conviction
is even a bigger key to success." —JNL

We know that focusing on what we want is essential in order to achieve it. But what happens if you don't know what you truly want? We must first work on gaining clarity. Getting clear about our goals and objectives in life is essential before we even start our journey. If we don't know what we want yet, that leaves us in a state of confusion. So we must achieve clarity first, above anything else. We must always have a crystal clear vision of what we want to achieve. If you're constantly confused, you won't get results. It's like going shopping for a new pair of jeans. You ask the sales lady to bring you a high rise cut in a dark wash, but before she brings it back, you change your mind to a low rise light rinse. If you keep changing your mind, you'll never actually get what you want in life. So get clear, by using my "1-2-3 Goal Setting Made Simple" formula.

How many times have you lost weight only to gain it back? How many times have you sabotaged yourself, treated your loved ones badly, and not taken care of yourself, only to say, "You know what? I'm not going fall back on these bad habits again"—only to repeat the negative behavior? How many times have you thought that just being skinny would make you happy, only to find out it didn't? It's because you didn't dig deep enough, and replace your hindering belief system with a helpful one—and you didn't have clarity with conviction.

Your Attitude and Belief Systems

Here is a metaphor to help us finally stop our bad habits, which actually stem from our inner belief systems. Many of us are raised to focus on the end result. We don't want to know how the clock is made; we only want to know what time it is. However, sometimes we need to actually look inside the clock to see why we are getting unsuccessful results in our lives. Our focus should be on enjoying the journey, not racing to the end result. Only by learning the lessons along the way to your destination can you get stronger, better, sharper, more resilient, and more determined to achieve your goals. This is where the band-aid approach must stop. We're going to get to the root cause; your attitude and belief systems.

Attitudes Are Contagious.
Is Yours Worth Catching?

"The problem is not the problem. The problem is your attitude about the problem." —ANONYMOUS

Some of us suffer from a bitter, negative, resentful, sour attitude. Having this bad attitude in life is harmful, as it steals your joy right out of your life, and it also trickles over to other people around you.

Do you think that shifting negative attitudes is a cinch to do? Remember, the number one spiritual tool to success is the Law of Gratitude. You can instantly flip any negative feelings or bad attitudes on their head by thinking of the things in your life that you are grateful for. In addition, when you combine your attitude of gratitude with positivity and optimism, it is inevitable that you will succeed.

This kind of super-charged, magnetic personality is essential in achieving a life worth celebrating. This attitude is like armor that guards your soul, which no unfavorable energy can penetrate. An optimistic, grateful attitude is priceless. It's like making huge deposits in your spirituality bank, allowing you to create beautiful memories and miracles in your life.

To increase the quality of your life, and to help you stay on the right track towards your weight loss and health success, aim to consciously keep a check on your attitude. Make sure you catch yourself if you feel your attitude becoming negative, and switch it instantly around by thinking of things in your life that you are grateful for. This is a powerful exercise which will produce wonderful outcomes in your life.

Improve the Universe by Improving Yourself First

"Place the oxygen mask on your face first,
and then assist those next to you."
— from the Flight Attendant pre-flight safety speech

Many are confused with what it means to be spiritual. Many see it as always putting themselves last. It is good to be unselfish to some extent; however, there comes a point at which, if you don't treat yourself with respect and love, you won't be truly happy. If you are always self-sacrificing, always giving to others and putting yourself last, your spiritual reserves will be in jeopardy. Yes, it is good to be helpful and kind. However, you must also be helpful and kind to yourself.

Here is a powerful metaphor. You are a holy temple. Your mind and your body are divine creations. Why would you ever put something dirty and of no value in such a sacred and special place? Why would you ever think unclean thoughts, entertain bad ideas, or even eat unhealthy food? You must also treat yourself with the respect and consideration you show for your loved ones. So start respecting yourself and treating yourself right, which will then provide an example and motivate others to do the same.

Remember the analogy of giving your best friend a fast food cheeseburger or a grilled salmon salad? Just like her, you deserve better than that processed fast food with little to no nutrient content. You deserve to enjoy an invigorating, life-boosting workout at least 4 times a week, to increase the quality of your life. If you've struggled with this, you're not alone. We've all been so conditioned to put ourselves last that we rarely feel we are worthy and deserving of the miracles a healthy lifestyle can provide for us.

Remember, you are the most important person in your life. If you can't help yourself, then how are you going to help others? It's like the airplane analogy. When you are on an airplane, in case of emergency, the flight attendant directs you to put on the oxygen mask first before helping others. This is the same principle with your health. This book is designed to help you first, so you are able to help others. Be a leader in your own life, so then show others how to be more resilient, self-sufficient, independent, ultimately victorious, and not a victim.

"I don't want to be thin and in shape. All of my fat friends won't like me." —a small negative inner voice inside all of us.

Some of you reading this subconsciously believe that it you start to look and feel fabulous, that your friends will start to be jealous of you, judge you, and talk about you behind your back. Yes, it's true; when you start using these timeless principles, not everyone will be super-happy that you are looking younger, radiating energy, and enjoying your newfound self-confidence.

> MBS DIET FIT TIP: Think about this: Does your staying in the rut help others? No, it doesn't. So get out of the rut, and embrace your new life, and never look back!

This is the breaking point. You need to continue on your new healthy path, and not allow your friends to hold you back from your true divine destiny. If they are true, unconditionally loving friends, they will be supportive of your new fitness program, and cheer you on. In addition, when you shine, you allow others to shine, too. You show them the route, the direction, and the pathway to their own personal successes.

If you feel that you may be slipping into some old unhealthy habits, take a good look at your "before" photo. Make it your aim to never allow yourself to go back to that old unhealthy lifestyle. Use your "before" photo as motivation to keep yourself moving in the right direction.

You Can't Help the Entire World— But You Can Help Yourself & Those Who Want to be Helped, Thus Inspiring Others

My own personal life coach taught me an invaluable lesson about not losing my focus and not wasting my energy. Here is a powerful metaphor to help you understand this Mind, Body & Soul Principle: You can't save a drowning person's life if you are drowning, too. So help yourself first by getting to solid ground and then help them.

I know this sounds a bit bleak and contrary to what I have been saying in this book. However, this is a very important principle. Let me prepare you for what is very foreseeable. You're going to find yourself on this great health kick, looking good, and feeling good. You're going to want to spread this message to the world. But you must be careful with whom you share your new found fitness knowledge. Some will want to hear what you have to say, and some will only want to criticize it.

This goes back to one of the most important lessons that Jesus taught us. In the Sermon on the Mount he preached, "Do not cast your pearls before swine." (MAT 7:6) This means, do not place what you hold sacred, important, and invaluable in front of those you know will have no respect for it. A lot of the other people around you are not prepared for this message of health, healing and happiness.

Sadly, some are not mentally, emotionally, or physically ready. They might judge you; they may try to discourage you. So, focus on yourself. Don't waste your time on people who don't have an attitude of gratitude. On the other hand, if you see someone who could benefit from these powerful Mind, Body and Soul principles, then share the light with them. There are so many who want to enjoy the pleasures of living a healthy, healed, and happy life once again. Be careful not to lose your focus in achieving your personal goals. If you are spending a lot of time and attention on those who are not ready, you won't have enough time or energy for yourself.

Accountability Matters

"The greatest thing a man can do in this world is to make the most out of the stuff that has been given to him. This is success, and there is no other."
—ORISON SWETT MARDEN, A.M, M.D.,
Author, Doctor, and Successful Hotel Owner

"Nobody can do it for you." —RALPH CORDINER,
Great American Business Leader of the 20th Century

A great lie that we are lead to believe is that we are entitled to a happy life, and that someone other than ourselves is responsible for making us happy. This notion could not be farther from the truth. The real truth is that there is one person to be held accountable for your life, and that person is you. It's plain and simple; if you want to be healthy, healed, and happy, it's all up to you. A big key to personal success in the Mind, Body and Soul Diet is taking 100% personal responsibility, and being accountable for your own life and your own outcome. You have the power to create, or remake the circumstances in your life.

Being 100% responsible for your life also means not blaming anyone else. You cannot play the blame game. We all have been conditioned from birth to blame everything and everyone other than ourselves, for our current state in life. We blame our parents, our work, the weather, the financial status of the world, our neighbors, our co-workers, our clients, and even our family for all of our disadvantages in life.

"When you stop playing the victim, you get out of the back seat, and into the driver's seat of your life, and in control of your destiny." —J N L

This also means that you have to stop, once and for all, playing the victim, stop blaming anyone else for your misfortunes, and give up all of your "poor me" excuses. For example, I could have blamed my "big body" Italian genes, falling back on the excuse that I have the "fat gene" in my DNA and that I would never be in shape no matter how hard I exercised or how little I ate. I chose not to play the victim, to own my destiny, and to take action. You can, too.

Focus on the solution, not the problem. This is a must-have mindset if you want to make the permanent transition from failure to success. It's nothing that I made up on my own. This is a universal truth which has helped millions before us become true successes in life.

We all can either choose to complain and talk about the problem, or we can choose to focus on creating a solution. Daily, make the conscientious decision to make the mental shift from focusing on complaining about the problem, to creating solutions. It takes less energy to focus on the solution, and you create an answer to solve your problems.

What happens when you focus on the problem? Your energy comes down. You become physically, mentally, emotionally and spiritually drained. You take your foot off of the ladder of success, and you place it on the rung of the downward spiral.

What happens to your energy when you focus on creating a solution? Your energy comes alive, you awaken your creative juices, and your mind goes into super-charged turbo mode, seeking for an answer to help you improve the quality of life. You feel more alive, and you are in more control of your destiny.

I once had a client named Ashley who came to me with a miserable outlook on life. It's as if her being overweight was directly correlated to her negative attitude in life. She was always the victim, blaming her unhappy childhood for her weight gain. She blamed her parents for not showing her how to eat right, and she blamed the food industry for making "diet food" more expensive. In her eyes, everyone was at fault except for her. Even though she was in her 40's and old enough to know better, she still didn't get the concept of taking full responsibility for her life. Her negativity was so charged that it almost seemed if she attracted all the weight to her body. She was so resentful that she had little to no self-love or self respect and her "fat suit" was like a protective guard telling the world to "stay away!"

I worked with her, week after week, month after month, reprogramming her old, outdated belief system that had convinced her that she had no control over her destiny and outcomes in life, making her understand that she had to give up all of her excuses. She is now more in control of her life, and uses her time wisely by not allowing life to just happen to her, but actually making the things that she wants to achieve in her life happen. She has dropped her anger, resentment and bitterness—and in the process, she also dropped her fat suit. Your negative emotions are linked to playing the victim, and so is your weight gain. Let go of them all so you may be your healthiest and best.

There is another side to this coin. Although we cannot always directly control some of the events in our lives, we can certainly control our responses to them. Don't let external limiting factors limit you! We stop ourselves from our own success because we focus on these so-called limiting factors. We have to get out of our own way, and stop blocking our path to our success by not allowing them to stop us. There is always a way around these obstacles. You must never take "no" for an answer when it comes to living out your dream life.

By choosing how we respond to what life hands us, we will have more direction in our lives, and more power in achieving our wanted outcome. You can change your thoughts, your choice of words, your decisions, and the visual imagery you have in your mind, in order to properly align them to your desired outcome.

The Consequences of Your Own Decisions: You Get What You Create

Here is a short and sweet example illustrating the two principles stated above:

Action: You have an extra hour in your day due to a meeting being cancelled.

Response: You decide to watch TV & eat junk food during the new-found free time

End Result: You feel sluggish, tired and bloated.

OR

Action: You have an extra hour in your day due to a meeting being cancelled.

Response: You decide to pop in an exercise DVD and work out

End Result: You feel invigorated, energized, and "thinner."

The Benefits of A Life Coach & Mentor

"People are not lazy. They just have impotent goals—goals that don't inspire them... by mastering a simple understanding of how your brain works, you can become your own therapist, your own personal consultant. You go beyond therapy, being able to change any feeling, emotions, or behavior for yourself in a matter of moments."

—TONY ROBBINS, *The Father of Life Coaching, Ranked by Harvard Business School Press among the "Top 50 Business Intellectuals in the World"*

MBS DIET FIT TIP: Life coaching is an emerging and rapidly growing field. A life coach is similar to a football coach who helps his players to develop, improve, and change to be the best. This is what I do, except in personal growth and development. If you are truly ready for real improvements in your life, then visit www.ClubJNL.com and apply for a one on one consultation with me. I can't wait to help you achieve your goals, as its my desire to awaken up your true passions in life-first helping you to realize them and then materialize them.

Becoming self-accountable will let you release the brakes that you've been putting on your success. If you can see now that what you've done in the past hasn't worked for you, this is where your new life starts. It's been scientifically proven that it takes approximately twenty-eight days, or four weeks, for a new, healthy habit to stick. Until you're ready to hold yourself accountable, hire a life coach to make you accountable for taking action and following through. A life coach is a nonjudgmental, third-party expert whose job it is to help you to see things of which you might otherwise be unaware.

A life coach will help you get from where you are now, to where you want to be, showing you the best, most fun, and most efficient direction. Your mentor will help you to constantly look in the direction that you are headed. Just like a financial analyst audits an account, you're going to audit your life to see if what you're doing is giving you results and if you are keeping your focus.

With our everyday demands and distractions, we are constantly derailed from our goals. This is where a life coach is extremely helpful, as they will help remind you of your vision and help you to get back on track and moving towards your goals. Remain flexible but also steadfast in your goal achieving. Implement the new tips, tools, and techniques I've provided you with, and understand that you can't control everything. However, you can get to the gym to work out, you can eat healthy, and you can get your rest. Stop focusing on things that you cannot control and always keep your eyes on the prize.

The Value of Community

"The people who you spend the most time with are the ones who directly impact and influence you the most-whether you like it or not." —J N L

When considering who the people are in your personal community, ask yourself this very empowering question: Does this person help me or hinder me in achieving my goals? The value of community is very much underestimated. Right now, take this quiz. On a sheet of piece of paper or right here in this book, write down the top five people with whom you spend most of your time. Then ask yourself honestly whether they help or hinder you in your personal growth.

1.

2.

3.

4.

5.

Now, regarding the five people named above, ask these questions:

1. Do these people know of my life's goals?

2. Are these people supportive of my new-found healthy lifestyle?

3. Do these people want me to truly achieve my goals?

4. Are they super-charged about my goals, pushing me to take action?

5. Do I feel that I can freely talk to these people, without fear of being judged?

Conclusion: If you answered "no" to many of these questions, then you can benefit profoundly through working with a super supportive, non-judgmental and knowledgeable life coach. Look in your area for a qualified life coach to work with, or log onto www.ClubJNL. com to apply to work with me one-on-one.

Energy Vampires are Good For Only One Thing: Sucking the Life Right Out of You

Have you ever had a conversation with someone that left you looking for the fang marks in your neck afterwards? You probably thought, "Wow, they just sucked the life right out of me." These people are energy vampires. Make sure you pinpoint the energy vampires in your life, and aim to limit your time around them. Here's a great method for steering clear of these energy vampires. When you see them coming, run the other way—or at least tell them you're busy and politely excuse yourself. Don't reply to their text messages, don't answer their e-mails, and don't take their phone calls. Stop sabotaging yourself by entertaining them when you know, in the long run, that you're only going to get the same result; you being more tired and drained.

On the other hand, have you ever met someone that inspires you, motivates you, and gives you energy? When you speak to them you actually leave feeling fuller and more effervescent. Add more of that type of person to your life. This is the power of community.

Take Veronica, one of my weight loss success clients, as an example. She has had a love/hate relationship with her mother for years; her mom meant well, but no matter what Veronica did, she was never good enough. In her mom's eyes, her husband wasn't good enough, her job wasn't good enough, her children weren't well-behaved enough, and Veronica was always being compared to her younger, "perfect" sister.

Veronica was emotionally eating because she'd never won the approval of her mother. This trickled down into her marriage and how she raised her kids—until I finally told her that it was okay to put herself on a "diet" from her mother. It was okay not to feel guilty if she took a little break from her mother, and it was time for her to realize that Mother doesn't always know best. More importantly, it was okay to give herself the gift of a valuable community of people who loved and supported her and didn't judge her.

I coached Veronica, as a grown, married woman and mother, that she must take one hundred percent responsibility for the life she is engaging in now, even if that means cutting back on the time she spends with her mother. By not allowing her mom into her personal space so much, Veronica gained more authority over her own life. It was a release for Veronica to come to peace with the idea that her mother was actually a hindrance to her personal growth and empowerment. That was a hard truth to swallow. Nonetheless, it allowed Veronica to heal, repair, and rebuild her life the way she wanted it.

Veronica told me, "This is the first time someone has told me that I am of full of worth instead of judging me. I feel like a big weight has lifted off of me." Since going on that little diet of time away from her mother, she had the authority back in her personal home and her mental space. She got back into the driver's seat of her life. She stopped letting her mom push her around, and as a result was able to lose weight. Her relationship with her husband moved to a passion level from 4 to a 10, thanks to putting the freedom back in their marriage. Veronica had more time to focus on her career, allowing her to become more prosperous financially because she wasn't being mentally and emotionally drained, and had the energy to be more involved in her work.

Seeing the miracles first-hand from taking control in her life, Veronica made the commitment to work with me once a month to continue the journey of her success. I helped her to build a circle of people around her that are supportive, not stifling; that are helping, not hindering; that are loving, not leeches; that are pleasurable, not parasites. She could not be happier or feel more free in her own life. She is an example of what a powerful life coach can do for you. If you feel imprisoned and not empowered in your own life, a life coach can and will help to liberate you.

If you don't know where to start, start with a life coach. Ask yourself, "Who can I lean on at this time to get me on an upward spiral?" You can visit me at JenniferNicoleLee.com and apply for a personal consult at www.ClubJNL.com. I can help you find the right contacts to start building that priceless community that will empower you, helping you to become the person that you were meant to be.

The Power of Congruent Alliances and Masterminding

"Organized effort is produced from the coordination of effort of two or more people who work towards a definite end in the spirit of harmony." —N A P O L E O N
H I L L from *Think and Grow Rich*

MBS DIET FIT TIP: Find people who you admire. Make a point to spend more time with them to pick up clues to their success. See what they do and initiate similar patterns in your actions and behavior. Some of the people who I most admire are authors, life coaches, and forward spiritual thinkers and healers. Therefore, I read their books, listen to their audio seminars, attend their seminars, and visit their websites. Find those who you look up to and can learn from, and do the same.

Make a commitment to surround yourself only with those who are loving and supportive of your life's goals. You will expedite your success by keeping worthy company. One of the principles of the Mind, Body and Soul Diet is to make a conscious effort to surround yourself with people who are in alignment with your new values and goals. Take another close look at the top five people you confide in, share your goals with, and also who you spend your quality time with. If they are hindering you, then find new relationships that will help you to achieve. You will quantum leap your results, and move that much more easily towards your desired objectives.

Remember, you can't have new people come into your life when other people are taking up that space. So make it a point, just like

Veronica did, to put yourself on a diet from unhealthy relationships that no longer serve you or help you emotionally, mentally, and physically.

Quality of Life

"The number on the scale does not represent your quality of life, nor is it equivalent to the dress size you wear. Rather, your quality of life is summed up by all of the different areas of your life, which are encapsulated in the mind, the body, and the soul." — J N L

People equate being thin, rich, and beautiful with happiness. This is only true to an extent. There is much more to joy. I know many people who are thin, rich, and beautiful, but who are miserable. Quality of life comes from being happy where you are right now, and then telling yourself that you can do better as you continue on your journey. Quality of life is measured in how much joy, peace, fulfillment, abundance, prosperity, health, wealth, happiness, and healing you have in your life.

MBS DIET FIT TIP: Being rich means you have money in the bank. Being wealthy means you have joy, peace, and true pleasure in your life and are full of love.

These days, we are living longer. If you're able to age beautifully, keep yourself mentally young and acute, and enjoy more energy and more excitement as you age, you will enjoy your golden years that much more. The great thing is, you're only as old as your mind, you're only as old as your body, and you're only as old as your spirit. That's why the Mind, Body and Soul Diet is designed to help you remain ageless, youthful, and disease-free.

"The growing recognition of the interconnectedness of body, mind, and spirit is excellent news for our society because it acknowledges that success begins with an integral approval. Ignoring any aspects of being causes a gap in one's ability to function harmoniously."

—MICHAEL BERNARD BECKWITH
author, *Spiritual Liberation*

The great thing about the Mind, Body and Soul Diet is that it's not a quick fix. It's a sound and balanced, holistic and whole-lifestyle program that addresses you as a complete person; mind, body and soul. I warmly invite you to visit www.MindBodyandSoulProgram.com, to listen to some of the testimonials that my students and fitness friends have shared. Not only have they lost weight, but they have also gained longevity through eating age-fighting foods and engaging in energy-increasing exercises. They have increased the quality of their relationships with themselves and their Higher Power, as well as with their loved ones. They have detoxed their minds and souls from the negative self-talk and belief systems that poison them. And they have shed their old skins to be reborn into their new, better selves. These are only some of the great advantages that the Mind, Body and Soul Diet will also help you achieve over time.

If you are like I was, silently suffering through emotional eating, finding comfort through food, yo-yoing with every fad diet and getting no results, you'll finally gain control over your health by eating the most delicious foods, doing the most exciting exercises, and for the first time, really, truly loving yourself as you are. It's going to be fun!

CHAPTER 9

Superfoods

"Eating healthy never tasted so good!"
—JENNIFER NICOLE LEE

W e are here at my favorite chapter—the chapter on food! I love food, and food loves me. That's the great part about the Mind, Body and Soul Diet; it isn't really a diet! We're going to plan our food, so let's call it a food plan, rather than dieting.

This is where you're going to stop eating accidentally and start eating optimally. You're going to eat foods that help you age gracefully, that actually have anti-aging properties to them, helping you to look and feel your best! You're also going to detoxify through eating the right foods. I'm going to show you how incredibly powerful food can be by giving you a list of JNL-approved super foods in this chapter, and super food recipes in the next.

"If you want to live a super fit lifestyle, then
you must eat super foods." —JNL

Super foods are defined as being nutrient-dense. That means they contain a lot of nutrients, minerals, vitamins, protein, and fiber, things that help your body run much more efficiently. These are foods you must eat daily, for energy and optimal weight loss, and to help you maintain mature muscle mass. And a great thing about the Mind, Bod and Soul Diet is that you can make this food plan a vegan or vegetarian one by substituting the lean meat suggestions for non-meat ones.

The Mind, Body and Soul Diet List of Super Foods:

Tea. I love to start with liquids because the body is made up of mostly water, and if you're not properly hydrated, your skin won't look good, your eyes will be dull, and you won't have a lot of energy. You should be constantly hydrating your body. So, make sure you drink water, but you can also have a tea party!

Tea has been around for ages. On my trip to China, all the beautiful teahouses amazed me. They drink tea five or six times a day and with every meal, which is part of the secret of their longevity. I was amazed by all the different kinds of tea: green tea, black tea, oolong tea, and white tea. Some were as expensive as my weekly grocery bill! However, you don't need to spend that much to get life boosting results.

Although green tea has a moderate amount of caffeine in its chemical makeup, it also keeps you hydrated. Green tea extract has a substantial effect on weight control, especially during the daytime. In addition to increasing your metabolism, the caffeine contributes towards a slight increase in energy as well. Most importantly, it's a great source of antioxidants. Plan to drink your tea with meals to increase your metabolism and keep you from eating as much. Healthy liquids keep you fuller in between meals as well. Try Lipton's entire brand line of high quality teas.

High fiber cereal. Fiber is your best friend in fighting and winning the war on fat, but very few people get enough fiber in their diet. Fiber also helps you detox, eliminate waste more easily, and feel fuller longer. High fiber cereals include steel cut oatmeal, which helps lower cholesterol. One of my personal favorites and one that I aim to have every morning is Kellogg's All-Bran Bran Buds Cereal. I top about ½ cup with blueberries and strawberries, walnuts, and drizzle with honey and add just enough skim milk to coat the cereal.

Wild fish. The key here is wild, not farmed. Farmed fish are encaged in their own waste. They also have higher levels of mercury, and just like adults and people who don't move around a lot, farmed fish are that much fatter and not as healthy. The best wild fish are salmon, mackerel, and sardines, which are high in the omega fatty acids vital for good brain function. Tilapia is amazing, too.

Bee pollen. Bee pollen is naturally rich in protein, vitamins, amino acids, and folic acid. Traditionally, it's been consumed to make the immune system stronger. It has over eighteen different amino acids, vitamins, calcium, copper, iron, phosphorus, potassium, fatty acids, carbs, and protein. If you suffer from seasonal allergies, try eating pollen from local bees. Bee pollen is really amazing; it even has a higher amount of protein than any other animal product. Also, the amount of amino acid in bee pollen is higher than that found in dairy products and meat. It has anti-aging benefits and should be used as a natural geriatric remedy. The pollen looks like little yellow specs and can be easily added to any recipe. Try topping your salad with it, stirring it into your salad dressing, blending it into your organic yogurt, mixing it into your morning oatmeal, or sprinkling it over your cut fruit for extra health benefits. Aim to take a teaspoon a day.

Lean red meat. Organic, grass-fed, lean red meat contains amazing vitamins and minerals you won't find in fish or even lean poultry: iron and vitamin B-12, as well as high amounts of protein.

Coconut oil. This is one of my favorites: organic, unrefined, virgin coconut oil. And if you don't believe me, then listen to this true story. In the early 1970s there was a surplus in coconut oil. It's very inexpensive, and farmers wanted to fatten their cows for prizewinning stock, so they tried feeding them coconut oil because it's very calorie dense and high in fat. The cows actually got leaner, more muscular, and had more energy and endurance.

Coconut oil stimulates the thyroid, thus stimulating metabolism, so you burn fat faster. Think about what this means. Healthy fat in, bad fat out—you need fat to burn fat. I like to put coconut oil in my fruit smoothies and protein shakes. I even pour it over my breakfast cereal. You'll find some great recipes in this book on how you can cook with coconut oil and use it as a condiment.

Finally, the same immune-boosting properties of lauric acid found in breast milk, are also found in coconut oil! What's the first thing that happens when you start losing weight on a diet? You get sick. So, if you are constantly getting sick, if you need to boost your immune system, take a tablespoon a day. On my very busy days, I take a tablespoon of coconut oil and blend it with a teaspoon of bee pollen. This is a nutrient dense super snack that is full of vitamins, minerals, and protein.

Nuts and seeds. Nuts are very healthy and nutritious. In addition to being excellent sources of protein, nuts and seeds contain many other benefits such as vitamins, minerals, fiber, and other chemicals that may prevent cancer and heart disease. Although many people are hesitant to eat nuts because they are high in fat, eating nuts can provide a sense of fullness and satisfaction that actually causes you to eat less of other high-calorie, high fat foods. Additionally, nuts are high in essential amino acids and healthy fats, making them an important part of any vegan or vegetarian's diet.

WHICH NUTS AND SEEDS ARE BEST?

Walnuts: The nickname of the walnut is the king of nuts. Look at it; it kind of looks like your brain. Curiously, it is actually really great for your brain. Walnuts are high in omega-3 fatty acids, which are essential for proper brain function, mental acuity, and focus.

Almonds: Almonds have cholesterol-lowering effects, also the ability to reduce heart disease risk due to the antioxidant action of the vitamin E.

Brazil nuts: Brazil nuts have been linked to preventing breast cancer, due to their high amounts of selenium.

Pistachios: High in iron, protein and fiber with high levels of magnesium, which helps to control blood pressure.

Peanuts: Not to be overlooked, this basic nut is an excellent source of B Vitamins, including folate, riboflavin and niacin, helping to reduce muscle degradation and fatigue.

Pumpkin seeds: Especially great for men to eat; they protect against prostate cancer.

Sunflower seeds: Rich in magnesium, which helps to regulate the nervous system.

Flaxseeds: Flaxseeds are especially fantastic. If you eat them whole, they act like little bristles to your intestines, keeping you more regular. Ground flaxseeds are also great because you can bake with them. Flaxseed oil is absorbed into your body quickly and makes an excellent addition to any protein shake or fruit smoothie. In Biblical days, oils (including flaxseed, primrose, and olive) were used as a healing topical to the skin; they were also ingested to heal. There's a certain mystery

behind the healing properties of oils, but one thing we do know—
they work!

Nut butters: This is a yummy way to eat your nuts.

....

Cayenne pepper: Cayenne pepper acts like a little windmill inside
your circulatory system. If you are on medication and feel like it's not
working, it's most likely because you've got poor circulation. Make sure
that you're including cayenne pepper in your food plan to help increase
your circulation and speed up your metabolism. If you have an adverse
reaction to hot, spicy foods, take a cayenne pepper capsule.

Pineapple: Fresh chunks of pineapple blended with water make a
delicious beverage and act as a natural anti-inflammatory to counteract
joint pain and swelling. It also contains a proteolytic enzyme bromelain, which helps in the digestion of protein. Pineapple can prevent
blood clot formation because of its bromelain content. My sons also
love this super sticky fruit and I use it in many of my protein shakes
and for juicing.

Blueberries: The number one super berry of all time is the blueberry, a natural antioxidant. Put it in your smoothies, on top of your
cereal, or just eat it plain. Blueberries will help you fight off the visible
effects of aging.

Sweet potatoes: Sweet potatoes are a staple of the Mind, Body
and Soul Diet. Sweet potatoes contain unique root storage proteins
that have been observed to have significant antioxidant capacities. They
are chock full of beta-carotene, vitamin A, and vitamin C. They're also
a complex, fibrous carb; so instead of pasta, which is a starchy carb,
have a sweet potato.

Brown rice: This is another staple carb of the Mind, Body and Soul Diet. It's good fiber and a great source of energy.

Cinnamon: This condiment tastes great and acts as a natural appetite suppressant as well. Put it all over your oatmeal, cereal, and mix into your coconut oil to put on your morning whole-wheat toast.

Asparagus: If you feel a little bloated, possibly from a high sodium meal the night before, asparagus is a natural diuretic. It's going to help you "pee off the pounds" and rid your body of water weight you're holding onto.

Ginger: In Eastern societies, ginger has always been known for its healing powers. It's known to heal and help motion sickness, help deter vomiting, and also help with migraines.

Red wine: As I've mentioned, this is one of my favorites due to its reduction of heart disease in women. So cheers to your health - salute!

Extra dark chocolate: It's chock full of antioxidants and helps boost your mood by releasing serotonin in your brain.

Apples: You can't go wrong with "an apple a day keeps the doctor away." It's high in fiber, and it fills you up. Have an apple before your meal and you'll eat less.

Celery: You burn more calories eating this detoxifying vegetable than not. It actually takes more calories to process the celery, so you burn fat while you eat.

Beets: I especially love to make juice with beets. See the section on juicing in this chapter. Red beet is unique for its high levels of anti-carcinogens and its very high carotenoid content. Red beets are high in carbohydrates and low in fat. It is an excellent source of folic acid. It is loaded with antioxidants that help the body guard against heart disease, certain cancers, especially colon cancer, and even birth defects.

Grapefruit: Grapefruit is an excellent source of vitamin C, a vitamin that helps to support the immune system. This glorious fruit is linked with flushing out fat from the body's system and also is super rich in antioxidants.

Fresh herbs: Seasoning dishes with fresh herbs is a superb way to raise the health benefits of any meal. For instance, parsley outstrips almost all other vegetables in its ability to raise the levels of antioxidants in your body. Cilantro helps to lower cholesterol. Find fresh herbs in your produce section, or grow some yourself at home.

Avocados: Avocados contain oleic acid, a monounsaturated fat that may help to lower cholesterol. Avocados are a good source of potassium, a mineral that helps regulate blood pressure. One cup of avocado has 23% of the daily value for folate, a nutrient important for heart health.

Cold pressed extra virgin olive oil: Pure, extra virgin olive oil is not only a light and delicate addition to many wonderful dishes; it is one of the most health-promoting types of oils available. Olive oil is rich in monounsaturated fat; a type of fat that researchers are discovering has excellent health benefits. Note: do not use for frying or sautéing as it produces toxic substances when heated. Rather, use it in cold dishes or drizzle over cooked food.

Tomatoes: Tomatoes contain large amounts of vitamin C, providing forty percent of the required daily value. They also contain fifteen percent of the required daily value of vitamin A, eight percent of recommended potassium, and seven percent of the recommended dietary allowance of iron for women and ten percent RDA for men. The red pigment contained in tomatoes is called lycopene, which is an antioxidant, neutralizing free radicals that can damage cells in the body.

Spinach: Spinach contains calcium, thus strengthening the bones. The A and C vitamins in spinach plus the fiber, folic acid, magnesium, and other nutrients help control cancer, especially colon, lung, and breast cancers. Folate also lowers the blood levels of something called homocysteine, a protein that damages arteries. So spinach also helps protect against heart disease. The flavonoids in spinach help protect against age-related memory loss. Spinach's secret weapon, lutein, makes it one of the best foods in the world to prevent cataracts, as well as age-related macular degeneration, the leading cause of preventable blindness in the elderly. Foods rich in lutein are also thought to help prevent cancer.

Bell peppers: Brightly colored bell peppers, whether green, red, orange, or yellow, are rich sources of some of the best nutrients available. To start, peppers are excellent sources of vitamin C and vitamin A (through its concentration of carotenoids, such as beta-carotene), two very powerful antioxidants. These antioxidants work together to effectively neutralize free radicals, which can travel through the body causing huge amounts of damage to cells.

Barley: Barley is a very good source of fiber and selenium, and a good source of phosphorus, copper, and manganese. It helps boost your elimination to keep you more regular, decreasing the risk of colon cancer and hemorrhoids. Necessary bacteria in the large intestine will also be increased by barley's dietary fiber.

Squash: Pumpkin, acorn, butternut, and spaghetti squash are in the winter squash group. Winter squash provide excellent sources of vitamins B1 and C, folic acid, pantothenic acid, fiber, and potassium, and carotenes. Look for richer colors as this denotes a higher concentration of these nutrients. Winter squash exert a protective effect against many cancers, particularly lung cancer. Diets that are rich in carotenes (especially pumpkins) offer protection against cancer, heart disease, and type-2 diabetes. Choose winter squash over summer since summer squash have a high water content; they are not as nutrient-dense as the winter varieties. However, summer squash still provide several nutritional benefits. They are low in calories and provide a decent amount of vitamin C, potassium, and carotenes.

Garlic: Garlic has long been considered an herbal miracle drug. Modern science has shown that garlic is a powerful natural antibiotic, albeit broad-spectrum rather than targeted. The body does not appear to build up resistance to the garlic, so its positive health benefits continue over time. The smartest way to eat garlic is taking it by supplement to avoid bad breath, or you can also cook with it to soften its flavor and odor.

Olives: Olives are a staple in the Mediterranean diet, known for their amazing health benefits. Olives are high in monounsaturated fats and are rich in vitamin E. Vitamin E is the body's main fat-soluble antioxidant, neutralizing free radicals in the body which are rich in fat. When monounsaturated fats are stable and the body has sufficient vitamin E, this adds to cellular processes like energy production. So grab a few olives a day by simply adding them to your salads, or enjoy with your anti-pasta dishes.

Horseradish: Due to its antibiotic properties, horseradish can cure urinary tract infections and kill bacteria in the throat that cause bronchitis, coughs, and related problems. I love it with my lean steaks for added health punch!

The Power of Juicing

*"Life is good! Squeeze every bit of
goodness out of it!"* — J N L

I'm here to tell you, as a health advocate and a fitness expert, that the typical two-week-long, extreme detoxing regimens just don't work to help you lose weight. When you go on a solely juice/vinegar/molasses concoction detox, you slow down your metabolism because you're not getting solid food, and you're hoarding the fat you already have. Your body senses that it's starving, so it holds onto your fat by slowing down your metabolism. Not only that, you're losing precious muscle tone and gaining more fat. So don't believe those twenty-one-day detox diet claims. Your body needs food to function.

I do, however, believe in juicing and drinking a glass every day with your food plan. It's a fast and efficient way to get amazing amount of vitamins and minerals that are easily assimilated into your body; plus, it's great for your kids. My sons love to watch how the juicer instantly pulls the juice out of an apple. It is beneficial and fun to work in a glass of fresh juice!

MBS DIET FIT TIP:
How Much Sugar?
I went to the grocery store and was absolutely amazed by how much sugar and carbs were in "juice" drinks—sixty grams of sugar in one can of juice! And these sweeteners are not natural. They are artificial and don't have anything near the amount of vitamins and minerals found in real live living fruits and vegetables.

THE ENDLESS BENEFITS OF DRINKING FRESHLY MADE VEGETABLE AND FRUIT JUICE

Let's face it, we all need to eat more fruits and vegetables. However, it's time consuming and difficult to prepare and eat our suggested daily servings. Juicing makes it easy to consume vegetables that are hard to eat, like spinach and even broccoli. And, speaking of vegetables, when you juice them with sweet oranges or apples, they just taste so much better, and are a lot more refreshing. Think about it—would you prefer to eat a bowl of steamed carrots? Or juice one with some apples and pineapple, and enjoy it in a tall glass over ice? That's the secret. Juicing is a way to deliciously "sneak" in more fresh fruits and vegetables. Consuming fruits and vegetables this way is just so much more pleasing. And here is the great thing; you can juice anything, fruit or vegetable! And the combinations are endless. You can get as creative as you want and have fun with it. Improve the quality of your lifestyle by juicing daily. And, trust me, there is nothing like a tall, cold glass of freshly juiced apples, grapefruit, oranges, carrots, lemons, pomegranates, blueberries, strawberries, beets, ginger, pears, celery, cucumber, and parsley… okay—you get the idea! Check my recipe section for great Mind, Body and Soul juicing recipes.

CHAPTER 10

Mind, Body and Soul Diet Food Plan and Recipes

T he main goals of the Mind, Body and Soul Food Plan are to nourish all three parts of the triad—the mind the body and the soul—to help you lose weight, gain strength, and to feel and look your best. Rule one; you must eat at least five to six times a day.

Breakfast: Start off with what should be both the most important and the largest meal of the day, breakfast. During sleep, you are at rest and, of course, not eating. And here is a hint: if you are waking up in the middle of the night to eat, then you are very off-balance. Therefore, when you awake in the morning it's vital to eat, in order to rev up your metabolism and stoke your fat-burning furnace. You will also be clear-headed and be able to think better with fuel in your body in the morning. Breakfast should be the largest meal of the day. In order to work with your metabolism instead of against it, make sure you trickle your calories down throughout the day, with dinner as your smallest meal.

Mid-morning snack: Around 10:30 or 11:00, it's important to refuel with a small mid-morning snack to keep your energy level high. Aim to consume around two hundred calories of a little protein and good-for-you

> MBS DIET FIT TIP: Make it a goal to not eat carbs after 4:00—you'll see major results! You can eat all the fibrous carbs (vegetables and salad) you want, but steer away from the complex carbs (brown rice and breads). You will wake up feeling thinner with more energy.

carbs. In the two-week sample menu, you will find quick, portable healthy snack ideas to eat on the go.

Lunch: Lunch should never be skipped! I always hear my clients state that they just can't break away from work to eat lunch because they don't have time or they don't feel hungry. I can't stress enough how important it is to eat lunch. If you skip lunch, you are setting yourself up to sabotage your food plan. You will end up eating more. You will also be more prone to eat high sugar and high carb foods later on. You're more likely to eat in the night if you skip lunch. Lunch needs to be a combination of lean protein, good-for-you whole grain carbs, a little heart-healthy fat, and fibrous carbs.

Late Afternoon Snack: Eating your late afternoon snack is like insurance. It will help you to not overeat at dinner and also keep your sugar levels even, so you don't binge later on. Eating a small, balanced two hundred-calorie snack around three or four o'clock will help you to keep your energy up,while helping you to not eat the whole grain carb at dinner.

> MBS DIET FIT TIP: One main reason for people eating heavy meals in the night is that they were "good all day," meaning they ate either too little or not enough. So make sure you concentrate on eating breakfast, your mid-morning snack, and lunch to insure you won't overeat at night.

Dinner: Dinner is a time to sit and relax with your family and friends. Value this time to eat together as a family and unwind from the busy day. Stick with your food plan, even if you see others are not, especially during dinnertime. The main focus here is to eat a lean source of protein with a heart healthy fat, along with some fibrous carbs, while staying away from complex carbs. Also, aim at only engaging in low-key, happy subjects to keep all negative or overwhelming

MBS DIET FIT TIP:
Have whole grain carbs
at lunch, but not at
dinner. If you are eating
a grilled chicken salad
for lunch, and then a
pan-seared fish fillet
with a sweet potato
and steamed asparagus
for dinner, switch these
two meals around. Have
what you typically have
for lunch for dinner, and
then what you have for
dinner at lunch. Your
lunch needs to be larger
in portion than your
dinner. Aim to have a
complex carb with lunch
during the day, and
to exclude it at night.
Making this simple
switch will help you
lose weight and to have
more energy during
the day, thus allowing
you not to hit that late
afternoon slump.

topics at bay, which could trigger an emotional eating splurge.

If you are still hungry after dinner, and you find that you can't go to sleep because of your hunger pains, quiet them down with a small low-carb, high protein pre-bedtime snack. I highly recommend a rich delicious protein shake made with water to satiate and quiet down your growling tummy. I prefer a pre-bed time protein shake because it replenishes my energy stores without causing me to gain weight, it hydrates my body because of its water base, and it also helps me to repair my muscle tone while I am sleeping. And the best part is that they are rich and delicious, almost like a good-for-you smoothie or "milk shake." Other healthy pre-bedtime snack options will be found in the two-week sample menu section.

Mind Body & Soul Diet Fit Tip: Remember the importance of eating five to six times a day. Take the small amount of time to "set yourself up for success" by pre-planning and preparing your meals ahead of time so you will stop eating accidentally.

Two-Week Sample Menu:

DAY 1

Breakfast—Eggs Florentine in a Warm Whole Grain Pita Pocket, recipe on page 188.

Midmorning Snack— Super Banana Split Protein Shake, recipe on page 216.

Lunch—Siciliano Protein-Packed Antipasto, recipe on page 198.

Late Afternoon Snack—Handful of unsalted nuts—blend of walnuts, pistachios & almonds.

Dinner—Cayenne Chicken Coconut Thai Soup, recipe on page 207.

Pre-Bedtime Snack—snack size cup of low-carb plain yogurt topped with fresh berries.

DAY 2

Breakfast—2 Kashi GoLean waffles, topped with sliced bananas and walnuts, drizzled with honey.

Midmorning Snack—Vanilla Coconut Protein Shake, recipe on page 193.

Lunch—6-inch Turkey Subway sandwich, with all the vegetables, snack size of crunch-pack apples, bottled water. (Hint: steer clear of the mayo, and you will make your lunch just that much healthier!)

Late Afternoon Snack—Twelve almonds with a small apple.

Dinner—Lemongrass Coconut Chicken Hot Entrée from Kashi.

Pre-Bedtime Snack—Small tin of tuna, rinsed, with a touch of fat free mayo & relish.

DAY 3

Breakfast—Blueberry Protein Pancakes, recipe on page 189.

Midmorning Snack—German Chocolate Cake Protein Shake, recipe on page 217.

Lunch—Barley Vegetable Salad with Feta, recipe on page 199.

Late Afternoon Snack—Snack size cottage cheese topped with sliced bananas, drizzled with honey.

Dinner—Grilled Grapefruit Marinated Chicken Breasts with Avocado, recipe on page 208.

Pre-Bedtime Snack—BSN's Fresh Cinnamon Roll Protein Shake—one scoop with 6-8 oz of water.

DAY 4

Breakfast—Egg white omelet with side of whole wheat toast.

Midmorning Snack—Super Berry Blast Protein Smoothie with Coconut Oil, recipe on page 193.

Lunch—Grilled chicken breast with sweet potato.

Late Afternoon Snack—Sliced banana topped with two Tbsp of almond butter with handful of whole grain pretzels.

Dinner—Grilled salmon breast squeezed with lemon, side of steamed asparagus and green house salad.

Pre-Bedtime Snack—2 hard boiled eggs with yokes removed, dashed with white pepper.

DAY 5

Breakfast—Southwest Veggie Omelet with a Side of Whole Wheat Toast, recipe on page 189.

Midmorning Snack—Key Lime Pie Protein Shake, recipe on page 217.

Lunch—Italian Turkey Meatballs, Sicilian Style, recipe on page 200.

Late Afternoon Snack—Small apple with 1 serving of string cheese.

Dinner—Roasted red peppers in olive oil with garlic shrimp.

Pre-Bedtime Snack—Strawberries and low-carb vanilla yogurt.

DAY 6

Breakfast—Plain fat free yogurt, swirl in 1 Tbsp sugar free preserves, ¼ cup Grape Nuts, and a tsp of local bee pollen.

Midmorning Snack—Coconut Cookies with a side of Fat-Free Cottage Cheese, recipe on page 194.

Lunch—Turkey & low fat swiss cheese sandwich on sprouted bread, small apple and bottle of water.

Late Afternoon Snack—Cut up crudités with drizzled hummus.

Dinner—Shake 'n Bake chicken breasts with broiled tomatoes, side green house salad.

Pre-Bedtime Snack—Small fat-free snack size cottage cheese with strawberries and blueberries.

DAY 7

Breakfast—Fortified French Toast Topped with Bananas Foster, recipe on page 190.

Midmorning Snack—Exotic Chai Tea Protein Shake, recipe on page 218.

Lunch—Oriental Beef Bowl with Stir Fry Vegetables Served Over Hot Brown Rice, recipe on page 202.

Late Afternoon Snack—2 Kavali 5-grain crackers and 2 table-spoons saba roasted eggplant.

Dinner—Baked Blackened Salmon Steaks with Mango and Black Bean Salsa, recipe on page 210.

Pre-Bedtime Snack—2 Quick Deviled Eggs—take 2 hard boiled eggs, slice in half, discard one yolk. Quickly mash the one remaining yolk with a little touch of fat free mayo. Top egg white halves with mixture, dash with black pepper.

DAY 8

Breakfast——Pizza for breakfast? Why not! Toast a split English muffin, top with 2 slices of tomato and low fat mozzarella cheese. Place under grill for a few minutes, and you have a nutritious breakfast.

Midmorning Snack—Winter Squash Soup with Slice of Swiss Cheese on Whole Grain Roll, recipe on page 195.

Lunch—Quick and Easy Cucumber & Turkey Sandwiches— spread 2 slices of sprouted bread with low-fat cream cheese, cucumber slices, reduced fat feta cheese, and a few slices of deli turkey for added protein.

Late Afternoon Snack—Slices of low-fat Swiss cheese on whole grain crackers with low sodium turkey slices.

Dinner—Grilled mahi mahi, with any of your favorite Mrs. Dash seasonings, with a side of sautéed spinach drizzled with olive oil and lemon.

Pre-Bedtime Snack—Chunks of cantaloupe wrapped in prosciutto.

DAY 9

Breakfast—Cottage Cheese with Exotic Fruits Drizzled with Coconut Oil, recipe on page 191.

Midmorning Snack—Cookies and Cream Protein Shake, recipe on page 218.

Lunch—Curry Chicken Walnut Cranberry Salad, Served Open Faced on Whole Grain, recipe on page 203.

Late Afternoon Snack—Small 6-inch, low-carb,whole grain tortilla with roast beef slices, rolled up.

Dinner—Succulent Exotic Asian Lettuce Wraps, recipe on page 211.

Pre-Bedtime Snack—Walnut and Strawberry Ricotta Whip—mix all ingredients together, drizzle with honey and enjoy: ½ cup of part skim ricotta cheese, ¼ cup walnuts, ¼ tsp almond extract.

DAY 10

Breakfast——Berry Blend—a cinch to make! 1 snack size cottage cheese, ½ cup of mixed berries—mix together and then top onto 2 slices of whole wheat toast.

Midmorning Snack—Chocolate Peanut Butter Supreme Protein Shake, recipe on page 196.

Lunch—Sunflower Seed Chicken Wrap—take one low-carb whole grain wrap, top with grilled chicken slices, black olives, sprinkle some sunflower seeds for extra crunch, spinach and diced tomatoes. Wrap and enjoy!

Late Afternoon Snack—Snack size cottage cheese topped with fresh blueberries.

Dinner—Quick and Healthy Sliced Beef Salad—cook steak slices, tomatoes, and purple onion together in a large skillet—douse it with a touch of balsamic vinegar and olive oil—top hot meat and tomatoes and onion mixture over a bed of greens.

Pre-Bedtime Snack—Four medium size precooked shrimp dipped in cocktail sauce.

DAY 11

Breakfast—Breakfast Burrito with Avocado on Whole-Grain Low-Carb Tortilla, recipe on page 191.

Midmorning Snack—Island Pina Colada Passion Shake, recipe on page 219.

Lunch—Tuna Salad in Pita served with Sprouts and Spinach, recipe on page 204.

Late Afternoon Snack—Nut Butter Toast with Crunchy Pears— toast 1 slice of sprouted bread, spread with nut butter, top with cashews for extra crunch, and then layer on slices of ripe pear. Drizzle with honey.

Dinner—Filet Mignon with Lemon Pepper Asparagus, recipe on page 212.

Pre-Bedtime Snack—1 wedge of Laughing Cow cheese and a handful of grapes.

DAY 12

Breakfast—"Speedy Gonzalez" Egg and Bean Tostada—whip up some egg white in a skillet, mix in some pinto or black beans, top with some low fat cheese and diced tomato—top this mixture onto a corn tostada. For extra fat burning—add a few hot chilis or a few dashes of Tabasco.

Midmorning Snack—Mochaccino Protein Shake, recipe on page 196.

Lunch—Quick Fix Barbecued Fajitas by Kraft—for a stress free fiesta, you can make chicken and vegetable fajitas. Use pre-cooked chicken tenders to save you time. In a large skillet sauté some sliced red bell pepper and white onion. Add about ½ Tbs. Kraft original barbeque sauce for added smoky flavor. Add chicken and cook for about 2 more minutes, until the chicken is well heated. Top onto whole wheat low-carb tortillas, like Tumaro's.

Late Afternoon Snack—Diced pear topped with walnuts and a dash of cinnamon.

Dinner—Maple and Mustard Glazed Salmon—mix 2 tablespoons of maple syrup and 2 tablespoons of coarse brown mustard. Coat salmon, and cook in broiler at 400 degrees until done. Serve with steamed asparagus with a squeeze of lemon.

Pre-Bedtime Snack—Apple Pie à la Mode Protein Shake, recipe on page 215.

DAY 13

Breakfast—Warm Walnut Cinnamon Apple Oatmeal, recipe on page 192.

Midmorning Snack—Chocolate-Covered Cherry Protein Shake, recipe on page 220.

Lunch—Chicken Tortilla Soup Topped with Avocado, recipe on page 204.

Late Afternoon Snack—Olive Cheese Melts—Take a toasted whole grain English muffin split in two, drizzle with cold pressed extra virgin olive oil, top with slices of tomato, fresh basil and sprinkle shredded low-fat mozzarella cheese and black olives. Broil for about one minute until cheese melts.

Dinner—Caribbean Shrimp and Mango Salad—easy to make and hard to resist; recipe on page 214.

Pre-Bedtime Snack—Turkey and Low-Fat Swiss Cheese Rollup— take 1 slice of carved sandwich sliced turkey breast and one slice of low fat Swiss cheese. Top the cheese on the turkey, and roll up. Optional—a touch of cranberry sauce, or even some course ground mustard.

DAY 14

Breakfast—Quinoa Cereal with Fresh Fruit. Top cooked quinoa with pumpkin seeds, sliced almonds, and your favorite berries. Mix in 1 Tbsp of coconut oil. Top with 1 Tbsp of bee pollen. Drizzle with honey.

Midmorning Snack—Low-Carb Flaxseed and Nut Granola Snack, recipe on page 197.

Lunch—Asian Turkey Burgers, recipe on page 213.

Late Afternoon Snack—The Turtle Shake, recipe on page 206.

Dinner—Shrimp & Avocado Salad—toss all ingredients and place inside a sliced open avocado: 1 cup cooked shrimp, 2 hard boiled eggs, ½ cup chopped celery, ¼ c. chopped green onions, ¼ cup chopped parsley, ½ c. chopped cucumber. ¼ c. chopped bell pepper, 4 Tbsp light Hellman's mayonnaise, 2 tsp hot sweet mustard, lemon and pepper to taste.

Pre-Bedtime Snack—Beautiful Berry Blast Protein Shake, recipe on page 215.

The Mind, Body and Soul Diet Recipes

When creating these recipes, I kept in mind the delicate balance of taste, ease of preparation, using Super foods, plus blending in antioxidant rich foods and heart healthy fats. Enjoy the pleasure of healthy foods again by making these simple, easy-to-whip-up meals. Re-awaken your "inner chef" by making it fun and including your children and family in preparing them.

Breakfast Recipes

EGGS FLORENTINE IN A WARM WHOLE GRAIN PITA POCKET

This is a healthy take on an old-time classic. Feel free to add sliced tomato.

Ingredients
- 1 cup fresh spinach
- Small clove of garlic, chopped
- 1 whole egg, 3 egg whites
- 2 Tbsp reduced fat feta cheese, crumbled
- Half of a whole-grain low-carb pita pocket

Directions
- Place a lightly coated nonstick pan with cooking spray over medium heat. Add garlic and then spinach. Sauté until it wilts. Whisk eggs until blended. Pour over the spinach, and cook to your liking. Top with cheese. Then place inside your pita for a quick yet filling breakfast on the go.

BLUEBERRY PROTEIN PANCAKES

I like to make these with my children. They love to add the berries. You can substitute the blueberries for any other berry you desire, or even use sliced banana. Sometimes I even replace the berries for chocolate morsels and make chocolate pancakes, to enjoy the healthy benefits of chocolate. You won't even need syrup on these because they will be so naturally sweet.

Ingredients
- 1 scoop of BSN's Whipped Vanilla Lean Dessert Protein Powder (to purchase, visit store.bsnonline.net)
- 2 egg whites
- ½ cup of blueberries

Directions
- Spray and heat skillet. Whip protein powder and eggs together. Pour batter onto skillet. Let one side cook while you add blueberries on top. Flip pancakes to cook the other side.

SOUTHWEST VEGGIE OMELET WITH A SIDE OF WHOLE WHEAT TOAST

Enjoy the health and beauty benefits of spinach, bell peppers, and eggs all in one super zesty dish. Serve with a side of whole-wheat toast for a complete energizing breakfast.

Ingredients:
- ¾ cups of your favorite veggies suitable for an omelet (I suggest spinach, onion, mushrooms, bell peppers)
- Touch of freshly minced garlic (optional)
- A handful of cherry tomatoes cut in half
- 3 egg whites, one whole egg

- Dash of black pepper
- Dash of cayenne pepper
- Sprinkle of shredded Mexican cheese

Directions
- Coat nonstick pan with cooking spray and place over medium heat. Whisk eggs. Add all vegetables and sauté. Pour eggs over into the pan and scramble lightly. Cook until done.
- Enjoy with a slice of low-carb toast.

FORTIFIED FRENCH TOAST TOPPED WITH BANANAS FOSTER

Making French toast with protein powder will keep you feeling fuller longer. Top with my healthier version of Bananas Foster for a breakfast you will be jumping out of bed for, and will never want to miss!

Ingredients
- 1 whole egg, 3 egg whites
- 4 slices of low-carb multi-grain bread
- ½ tsp of cinnamon
- 1 scoop of BSN's Fresh Cinnamon Roll Lean Dessert Protein Powder
- Topping: One sliced banana, 2 Tbsp maple syrup.

Directions
- Whisk the eggs together in a medium size bowl. Add the protein powder and stir until smooth. Add cinnamon to mixture. Dip the bread, thoroughly coating each side. Spray a nonstick skillet with cooking spray and place on medium heat. Place the protein-coated bread into the frying pan. Cook until golden brown about three minutes.

□ Topping: lightly coat a small nonstick skillet with butter-flavored cooking spray and place over medium heat. Add sliced bananas and fry for about one minute.

TROPICAL COTTAGE CHEESE WITH EXOTIC FRUITS DRIZZLED WITH COCONUT OIL

This is a great breakfast to whip up when you are in a hurry. It's tropical in flavor and texture because of the sweet pineapple and coconut oil.

Ingredients
□ Small snack-size portion of cottage cheese

□ Fruit of your choice, try blueberries or pineapple

□ 1 tsp of bee pollen

□ Whole grain English muffin

□ 1 Tbsp of coconut oil

Directions
□ Toast English muffin. Blend bee pollen and fruit into cottage cheese. Top English muffin with mixture. Drizzle with coconut oil on top.

BREAKFAST BURRITO WITH AVOCADO ON WHOLE-GRAIN LOW-CARB TORTILLA

Wake up your taste buds in the morning with this meal that sends your mouth on a vacation south of the border! You will make your mouth say "Ole!"

Ingredients
□ 1 8-inch whole-wheat low-carb tortilla

□ 1 whole egg, 3 egg whites

□ ¼ cup black beans or pinto beans

- Sprinkle of shredded reduced fat Mexican cheese
- One small tomato, diced
- Half of one small avocado

Directions
- Lightly coat a nonstick skillet with cooking spray. Place over medium heat. Warm up the tortilla by placing it in skillet, turning over after thirty seconds on each side. Set aside.
- Beat eggs and pour into skillet. Cook until done, then add to skillet your tomato, beans, and cheese. Put eggs onto warmed tortilla and then top with avocado. Fold tortilla and enjoy.

WARM WALNUT CINNAMON APPLE OATMEAL

Start your day off right with a hearty breakfast, full of rich texture that will stick to your ribs! The added protein powder will fortify your warm cereal with protein for a balanced breakfast.

Ingredients
- ½ cup of instant oatmeal
- 1 cup of hot water
- 1 scoop of BSN's Lean Dessert Protein Powder Fresh, Cinnamon Roll Flavor
- Small apple, cored and sliced into wedges
- 1 Tbsp of coconut oil
- ¼ cup of walnuts
- Dash of cinnamon

Directions

- In skillet, warm up coconut oil and place apple wedges and walnuts in pan. Add a dash of cinnamon. Cook for about three minutes until apples get soft. In a bowl place oatmeal and water. Place in microwave for thirty seconds, stirring when done. Top with apples and walnut mixture.

Midmorning Snacks

VANILLA COCONUT PROTEIN SHAKE

Ingredients

- One scoop of BSN's Lean Dessert Protein Powder, Whipped Vanilla Flavor
- 1 Tbsp of coconut oil
- 1 tsp of bee pollen
- 1 Tbsp of ground flax seed
- 1 Tbsp of coconut flakes (optional)
- 3 cubes of ice
- 8 ounce of water
- Blend and enjoy.

SUPER BERRY BLAST PROTEIN SMOOTHIE WITH COCONUT OIL

Vitamin C and photochemical rich sweet berries, swirled into your creamy vanilla shake with an essence of tropical coconuts—this power drink will send you into heaven!

Ingredients

- One scoop of BSN's Lean Dessert Whipped Vanilla Protein Powder
- ½ cup of mixed berries (strawberries, blueberries, raspberries, blackberries)
- 1 tsp of bee pollen
- 1 Tbsp of ground flaxseed
- 3 cubes of ice
- 8 ounce of water
- Blend and enjoy

COCONUT COOKIES WITH SIDE OF FAT FREE COTTAGE CHEESE

They sound sinful, but they're not! They are actually great for you because they are low in sugar, high in fiber, and the flaxseeds add texture and are a great source of essential fatty acids. What a great, guilt-free energy boosting treat! Enjoy with a snack-size fat-free cottage cheese.

Ingredients

- 1 cup unsweetened coconut flakes
- 3 Tbsp warm water
- 1 whole egg
- 1 Tbsp honey
- 1 tsp coconut oil
- ¼ cup flaxseeds
- 1 cup old-fashioned oats

Directions

- Mix warm water and honey together. Add coconut flakes. Beat in the egg. Mix thoroughly. Form into balls and drop by spoonful on well-greased cookie sheet. Bake at 400 degrees for twelve to fifteen minutes.

WINTER SUPER SQUASH SOUP WITH SLICE OF SWISS CHEESE ON WHOLE GRAIN ROLL

Squash is loaded with vitamin C (great for boosting your immune system and to fight off colds) and fiber (to keep you regular). The cayenne is great for circulation, and the coconut oil has medicinal properties to fight off infections and stimulate the thyroid. But you won't even think of this soup as your typical "healthy meal" because of how rich and satisfying it is!

Ingredients
- ¾ Spanish onion
- Small clove of garlic, minced, or use minced garlic in jar
- 2 tsp coconut oil
- 2½ tsp curry powder
- 1 dash of cinnamon
- ½ tsp cayenne pepper
- 4 cups reduced sodium non-fat chicken or vegetable broth
- 5 large winter squash, baked until soft
- 1 sweet potato, baked until semi-soft then cubed
- Dash of black pepper
- Topping: fat free sour cream and whole-wheat croutons

Directions
- In large saucepan, sauté onion and garlic. Add black and cayenne pepper, stirring to coat. Add broth, sweet potatoes, squash, and bring to a boil. Reduce heat to medium, partially cover, and cook for about seven to ten minutes. Remove from heat, top with a dollop of sour cream and whole wheat croutons.

CHOCOLATE PEANUT BUTTER SUPREME PROTEIN SHAKE

Satisfyingly thick, rich, and super creamy, this shake will stop hunger in its tracks without blowing your food plan.

Ingredients

- 8 ounces of cold water
- One scoop of BSN's Lean Dessert Protein Powder, Chocolate Fudge Pudding Flavor
- 1 Tbsp natural no sugar added/no trans fat peanut butter
- 3 ice cubes

Directions

- Blend and enjoy!

MOCHACCINO PROTEIN SHAKE

I usually make this with leftover cold coffee that is left in the pot from breakfast. Or you can use instant coffee instead. It's an energy booster that's rich and creamy!

Ingredients

- One scoop of BSN's Syntha 6 Mochaccino Flavored Protein Shake Powder
- 8 ounces of cold water
- ¼ cup of cold coffee or 2 tsp of instant coffee granules

Directions

- Blend and Enjoy!

LOW-CARB FLAXSEED AND NUT GRANOLA

A treat I created that my entire family loves whip up together and eat!

Ingredients
- 1 cup flaxseed
- 1 cup sunflower seeds, unsalted
- 1 cup unsweetened shredded coconut
- 1 cup each chopped pecans, walnuts, and almonds
- ½ cup of coconut oil, melted
- 2 tsp cinnamon
- 2 tsp BSN Lean Dessert Protein Powder, Whipped Vanilla Flavor

Directions
- In a large roasting pan, mix the flaxseeds, sunflower seeds, coconut, and nuts. Drizzle with the melted coconut oil. Stir in cinnamon, vanilla protein powder. Toast in the oven at 325 degrees for thirty minutes. Stir every five to ten minutes.

Mind, Body and Soul Diet Fit Tip: This recipe gives you six servings. I suggest you prepare and then portion out into six plastic sandwich bags for a portable treat to take on the go.

Lunch Recipes

SICILIANO PROTEIN-PACKED ANTIPASTO

Being Italian, my parents frequently prepared a large platter of delicious cheeses, meats, veggies, and olives. This dish makes for an interesting and fun lunch that is just as pleasing to the eye as it is to the tummy! Here is my healthy version in honor of them.

Ingredients
- Lean cuts of sliced turkey breast, roast beef, and prosciutto
- Black and green olives, rinsed off to remove excess salt
- Low fat Swiss cheese
- Low fat mozzarella cheese
- Cherry tomatoes cut in half
- Broccoli florets and carrot sticks
- Dash of minced fresh Italian herbs such as oregano, basil, parsley, sage, or rosemary
- Whole wheat bread

Directions
- On a plate, beautifully arrange all the ingredients for a delectable presentation.

Mind, Body and Soul Diet Fit Tip: Rinse the olives and meats with cold water to remove unnecessary salt. Feel free to drizzle the veggies with olive oil for an extra added health benefit.

BARLEY VEGETABLE SALAD WITH FETA

Hands down, barley is one of the best whole grains for you because it carries more fiber than brown rice. Barley is also high in viscous soluble fiber, which helps to lower LDL cholesterol, the so-called "bad" cholesterol, thus reducing the risk factor of heart disease. Barley is usually used in soups or stews but I like to use it to "beef" up a delicious vegetable salad sprinkled with feta. Dig in with no guilt!

Ingredients
- 1 cup cooked hulled barley
- 1 cup water
- 1 green or red bell pepper, seeded and diced
- 1½ cups chopped carrots
- 1 cup red cabbage
- ½ cup minced red onion
- ¼ cup minced sundried tomatoes
- 1 Tbsp red wine vinegar
- 2 tsp creamed horseradish
- 1 tsp olive oil
- Coarsely ground black pepper to taste
- Dash of cayenne pepper
- 2 Tbsp of feta cheese (optional)

Directions
- Cook hulled barley. Put in large mixing bowl; add green or red bell pepper, carrots, cabbage, tomatoes, and onion. In a small bowl, mix together vinegar, horseradish, and oil. Pour over barley mixture and stir to coat. Top with feta cheese. Season with black and cayenne pepper.

Mind, Body and Soul Diet Tip: This is an excellent zesty vegetarian salad. Feel free to omit the feta if you are on a vegan diet. Also, the horseradish in this dish helps to fight off colds and clears your sinuses if you are congested.

ITALIAN TURKEY MEATBALLS, SICILIAN STYLE

One of my favorite childhood memories was warming up with a big bowl of homemade spaghetti and meatballs. Here is my modern day version. I traded out the ground beef for low fat turkey, slashing the calories while keeping the protein high. As for the pasta, use whole wheat or spinach pasta to up the fiber. Yes, you can have carbs, but the right ones. Enjoy one cup of pasta and two meatballs to keep in line with your portion control. And as we say in Italian, *mangi*!

Ingredients
- Cooking spray
- 1 lb antibiotic-free ground turkey
- 1 slice whole wheat bread, crust removed pulsed into crumbs
- ¼ cup grated Parmesan
- ½ grated carrot
- 2 large cloves of garlic, minced
- 2 Tbsp minced parsley
- 2 tsp minced fresh thyme leaves
- 1 egg lightly beaten
- ½ teaspoon salt
- Freshly ground black pepper
- 1 box whole wheat pasta

Directions

▫ In a 4-quart saucepan heat the oil over medium heat. Sauté the onions until translucent, about three minutes, then add the garlic and cook for one minute more. Add tomato paste, tomatoes, oregano, rosemary, and salt. Bring all the ingredients to a low boil, reduce heat and cook for approximately fifteen minutes, until liquid has evaporated slightly. Season with salt and pepper, to taste. While sauce is cooking, make meatballs. Preheat the broiler. Spray a baking sheet with cooking spray. Combine the turkey with all other ingredients, except for the fresh basil, in a large work bowl. Form into two and a half inch balls and place on a baking sheet. Broil for ten minutes, or until browned and almost entirely cooked through. Meanwhile, remove rosemary sprig from sauce and add fresh basil. Add the meatballs to the sauce, cover, and cook an additional ten minutes, or until sauce has slightly thickened and meatballs have absorbed some of the sauce. While the meatballs are cooking, cook the whole wheat spaghetti according to package directions.

▫ Drain the pasta and return it to the pot. Add the sauce and meatballs, toss and heat through over medium heat. Divide evenly among four pasta bowls and garnish with parsley and one tablespoon grated Parmesan.

ORIENTAL BEEF BOWL WITH STIR FRY VEGETABLES OVER HOT BROWN RICE

Take a trip to the Orient with this exotic and succulent recipe. Don't let its complexity fool you, as it's a cinch to prepare.

Ingredients
- 1 pound beef flank steak, well-trimmed
- 2 Tbsp Oriental dark-roasted sesame oil, divided
- 2 Tbsp reduced-sodium soy sauce
- 1½ tsp raw brown sugar
- 1 tsp cornstarch
- ¼ tsp crushed red pepper pods
- 2 cloves garlic, crushed
- 1 Tbsp fresh ginger, minced
- 1 small red pepper cut into 1" pieces
- 1 small can whole baby corn
- 4 ounces snow pea pods, julienned
- 2 Tbsp chopped parsley

Directions
- Partially freeze beef flank steak to firm (approx. 30 minutes). Cut steak in half lengthwise; cut each half across the grain into eighth-inch strips. Combine one Tablespoon sesame oil, soy sauce, sugar and cornstarch; pour over beef strips, tossing to coat. Heat remaining sesame oil in wok or large nonstick skillet over medium-high heat. Add pepper pods, garlic and ginger; cook thirty seconds. Add pepper and corn; stir-fry ninety seconds. Add pea pods; stir-fry thirty seconds. Remove vegetables from pan; reserve. Stir-fry beef strips (half at a time) two to three minutes. Return vegetables and

beef to pan and heat through. Top with fresh parsley for added antioxidants.

Mind, Body and Soul Diet Fit Tip: Invest in a rice cooker, which will help you to always have a healthy complex carb on hand without the cooking. You simply add water and brown rice, and shut the lid. The cooker will prepare brown rice and keep it fresh for at least three days.

CURRY CHICKEN WALNUT CRANBERRY SALAD, SERVED OPEN FACED ON WHOLE GRAIN

Make over your old-fashioned chicken salad with my new innovative version that has added crunch from the celery and walnuts. Make this batch large to save for leftovers.

Ingredients
- 4 large skinless boneless chicken breasts, cooked and diced
- 1 stalk celery chopped
- 1 small apple, cored and cut into small chunks
- 1 cup seedless red grapes
- ½ cup walnuts
- Dash of white pepper
- ½ teaspoon of curry powder
- ¾ cup light or fat free mayonnaise
- ½ cup dried cranberries

Directions
- In a large salad bowl combine the chicken, celery, onion, apple, cranberries, grapes, walnuts, pepper, curry powder, and mayonnaise. Mix all together, tossing to

coat. Salad is ready to serve with your toasted whole wheat roll. Feel free to add a slice or two of tomato and some fresh spinach leaves to up your vitamins and antioxidants to this meal.

TUNA SALAD IN PITA SERVED WITH SPROUTS AND SPINACH

Ingredients
- ½ cup chopped red pepper
- ¼ cup bottled pickled vegetables, drained and chopped
- ¼ cup finely chopped red onion
- ¼ cup fat-free mayonnaise
- 1 (12-ounce) can albacore tuna in water, drained and flaked
- 2 tsp fresh minced parsley
- 2 cups of spinach
- Alfalfa sprouts

Directions
- Combine the first six ingredients in a medium bowl. Scoop a half cup tuna salad into four pitas. Top each with spinach and a few threads of alfalfa sprouts.

CHICKEN TORTILLA SOUP TOPPED WITH AVOCADO

Full of low fat protein, essential fatty acids (EFAs) from the avocado and the citrus punch of the lime make this soup a show-stopper.

Ingredients
- 3 medium-sized cans of fat-free chicken broth
- ½ bunch of washed and chopped cilantro
- 1-2 ripe avocados peeled and sliced into small chunks

- 3 tiny pinches of thyme
- 1 pinch of marjoram
- 1 Tbsp of onion
- 1 block of skimmed mozzarella cheese (80 calories per ounce)
- Whole grain tortilla chips
- 2 small limes, seeded and diced into wedges
- 1 small package of chicken tenders
- White pepper, if desired
- Dash of cayenne

Directions

- Empty the chicken broth and chopped cilantro into a large kettle or pot, adding two cans of water, the onion, thyme, and marjoram. Cook on medium heat. Spray a skillet or pan with nonstick cooking spray and cook chicken slowly so that it caramelizes on both sides. When chicken is done, cut into bite-sized chunks and transfer to the broth. Cook until hot but not bubbly. Toss in the diced, seeded limes, leaving on the rinds. The rinds add a citrus punch to the soup, plus the soup will have a more exotic presentation. Top each bowl with crushed up tortilla chips, the avocado and a sprinkle of cheese.

Mind, Body and Soul Diet Fit Tip: Coat the chunked avocado with some of the lime juice to prevent browning.

Late Afternoon Snack

- Twelve almonds with a small apple
- Sliced banana topped with two tablespoons of almond butter, with handful of whole-grain pretzels
- Cut up crudités with hummus
- Slices of low-fat Swiss cheese on whole grain crackers with low sodium turkey slices
- Snack-size fat-free cottage cheese topped with fresh blueberries
- Diced pear topped with walnuts and a dash of cinnamon

THE TURTLE SHAKE

One of my favorites, this whimsical take on the famous chocolate, pecan, and soft caramel treat is impossible to resist!

Ingredients

- 1 scoop BSN Lean Dessert Protein Shake, Chocolate Fudge Flavor
- 1 ounce pecan halves, chopped
- 2 Tbsp natural peanut butter
- 3 ice cubes
- 1 Tbsp sugar-free and fat-free caramel syrup
- Blend and enjoy!

Dinner

CAYENNE CHICKEN COCONUT THAI SOUP

It's known that soup fills you up, thus quickly cutting your appetite. Make a whole pot, and freeze individual portions. You can also bring this soup with you to work and warm it up in the microwave for a hot, delicious snack that will fill you up—and not with guilt! It's also a great soup to make if you feel a cold coming on. The cayenne helps to fight off fever, and the coconut oil boosts your immune system.

Ingredients
- 1 tsp coconut oil
- 1 Tbsp unsalted butter
- 1 clove garlic chopped
- 4 shallots, chopped
- 2 small fresh red chili peppers, chopped
- 1 cup red pepper, sliced lengthwise
- 1 cup broccoli
- 1 Tbsp chopped lemongrass
- 2½ cups chicken stock
- 6 ounces lean chicken breast cut into bite size chunks
- 1½ cups unsweetened coconut milk
- 1 bunch fresh basil leaves

Directions
- In a medium saucepan, heat oil and butter. Sauté the garlic, shallots, chilies, red pepper, broccoli, and lemongrass in oil until fragrant. Stir in chicken stock, coconut milk, and bring almost to a boil. Simmer on low heat until chicken is cooked. Add some cayenne at

this point. Make it as hot and spicy as you like. You can go wild or mild, it's your choice!

GRILLED GRAPEFRUIT MARINATED CHICKEN BREASTS WITH AVOCADO

Bored with chicken? Well, not with this recipe!

Ingredients
- 4 boneless and skinless chicken breasts
- 1 pink grapefruit
- 1 navel orange
- Lemon pepper seasoning
- One whole avocado sliced

Directions
- Marinate the chicken breasts overnight in a mixture of freshly squeezed grapefruit, lemons, and oranges. Sprinkle with lemon pepper. Coat a medium sized nonstick pan with cooking spray, place on medium heat. Cook through. Take out of pan. Place the four slices of grapefruit in pan; cook until warm both sides. Top chicken with grapefruit slices and sliced fresh avocado.

ROASTED RED PEPPERS IN OLIVE OIL WITH GARLIC SHRIMP

Peppers are powerhouses packed with an incredible amount of vitamin C, giving you almost 300% of your RDA per serving. Shrimp is an excellent source of low fat, low calorie protein, which is also high in selenium. Not to mention that everyone knows the wonders of olive oil and garlic!

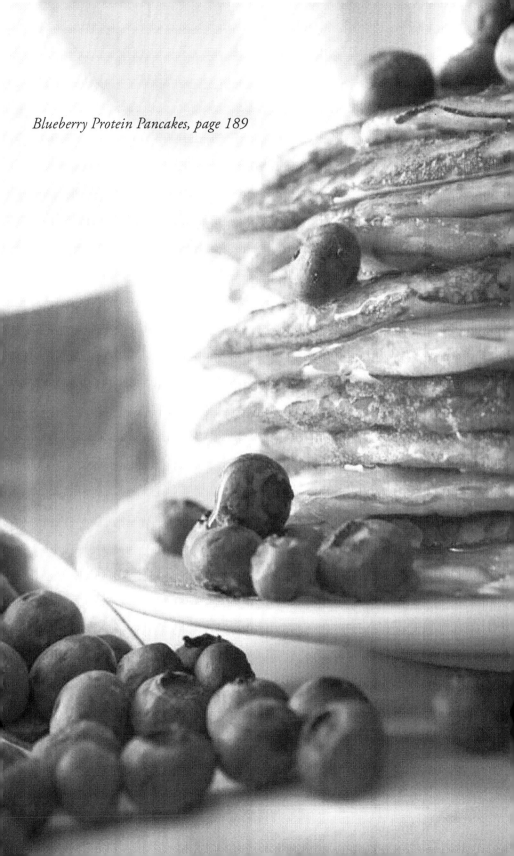

Blueberry Protein Pancakes, page 189

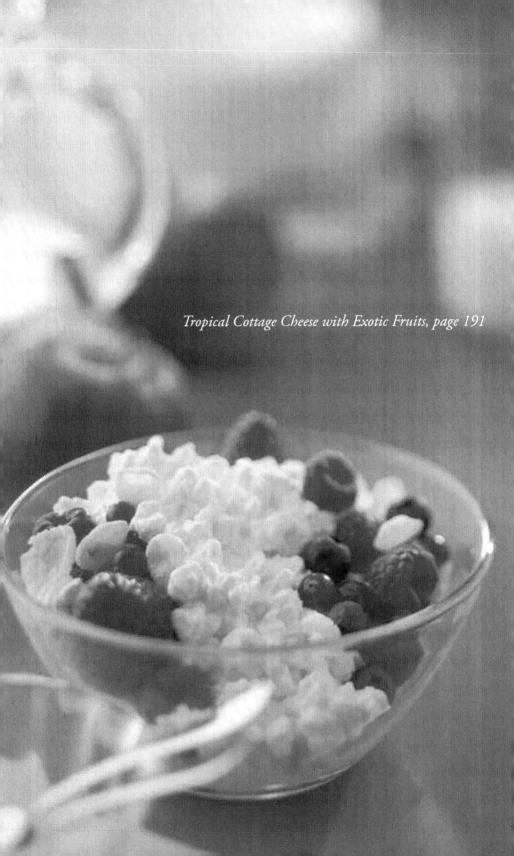
Tropical Cottage Cheese with Exotic Fruits, page 191

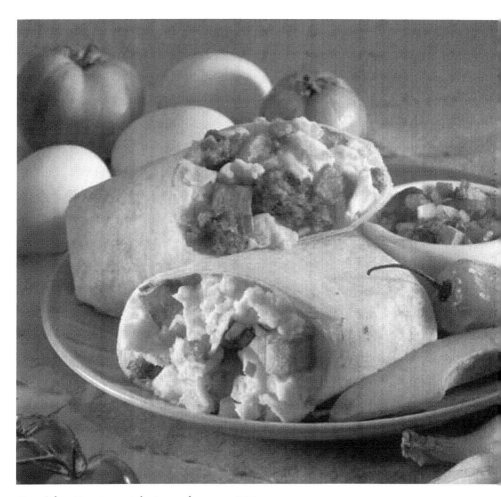

Breakfast Burrito with Avocado, page 191

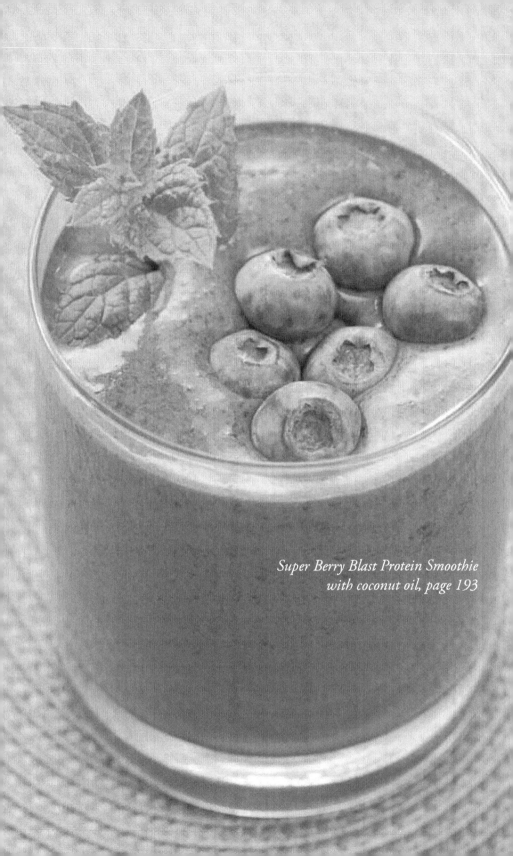

*Super Berry Blast Protein Smoothie
with coconut oil, page 193*

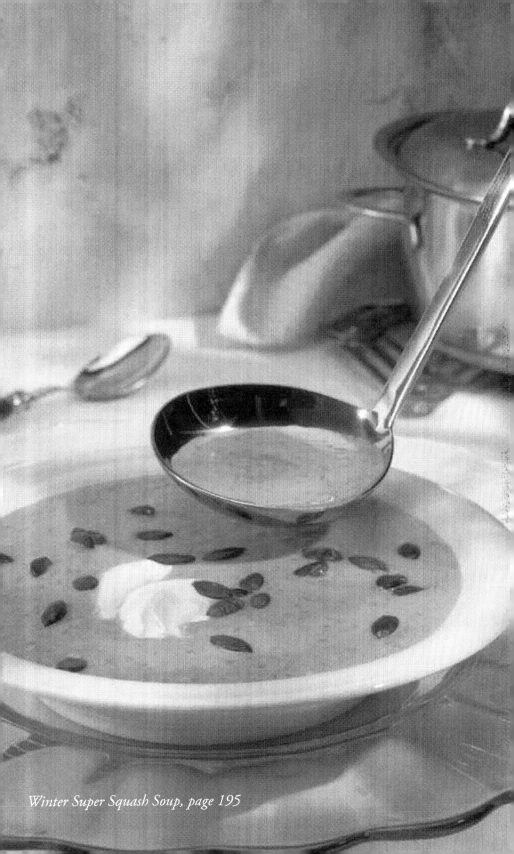

Winter Super Squash Soup, page 195

Mochacinno Protein Shake, page 196

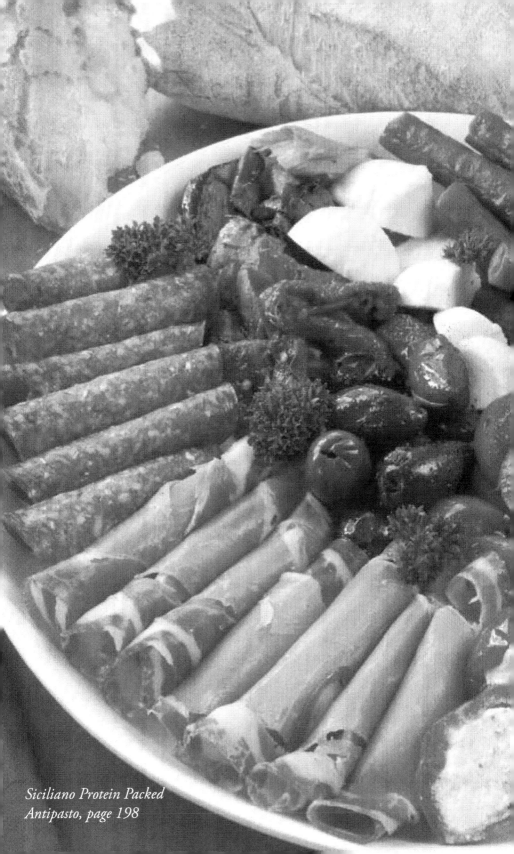

Siciliano Protein Packed
Antipasto, page 198

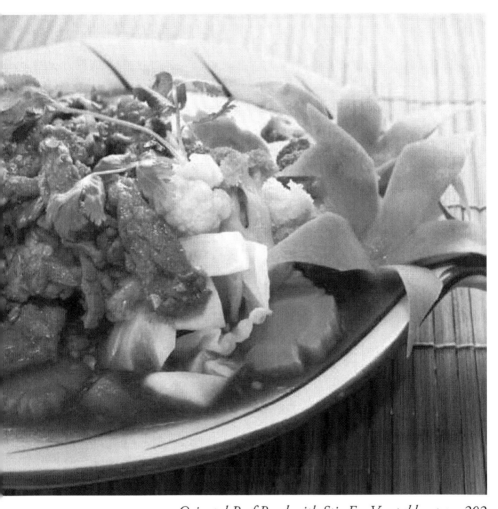

Oriental Beef Bowl with Stir Fry Vegetables, page 202

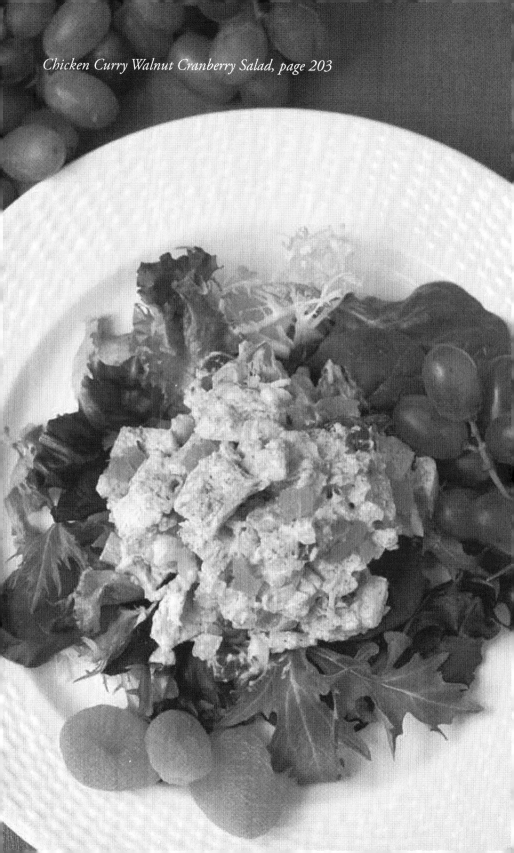

Chicken Curry Walnut Cranberry Salad, page 203

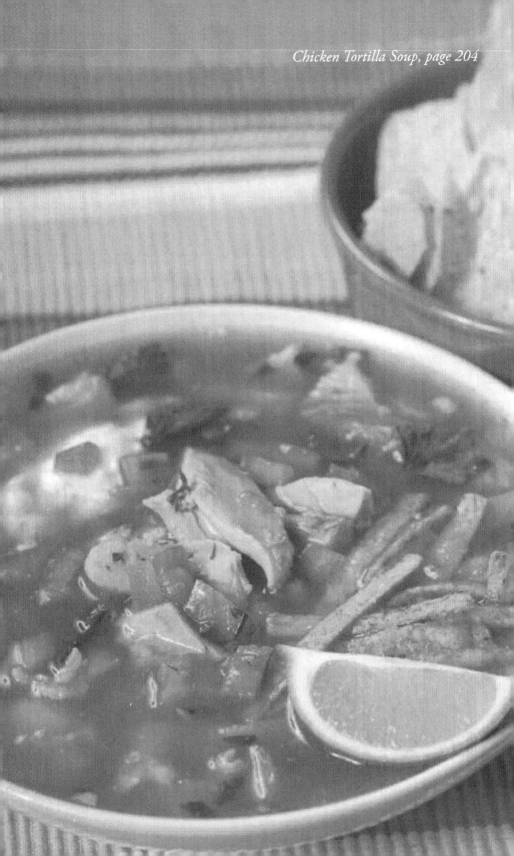

Chicken Tortilla Soup, page 204

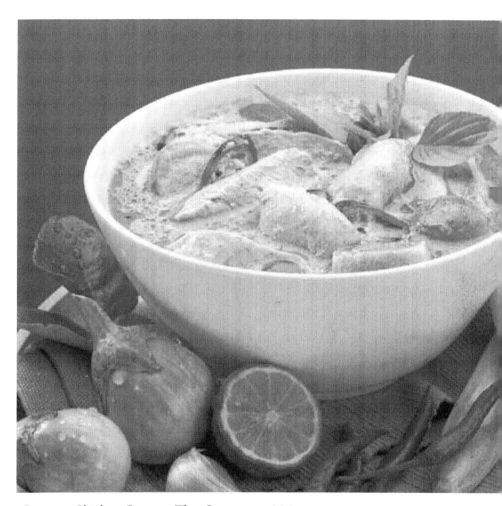

Cayenne Chicken Coconut Thai Soup, page 207

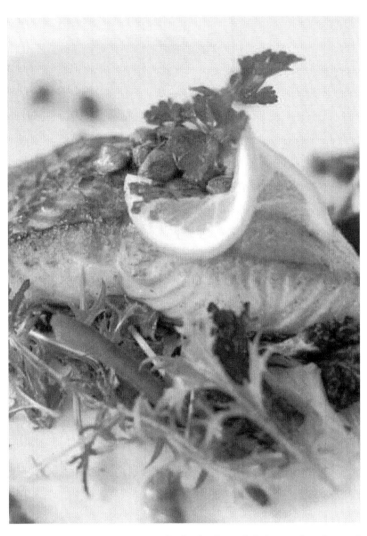

Baked Blackened Salmon Steaks with
Mango and Black Bean Salsa, page 210

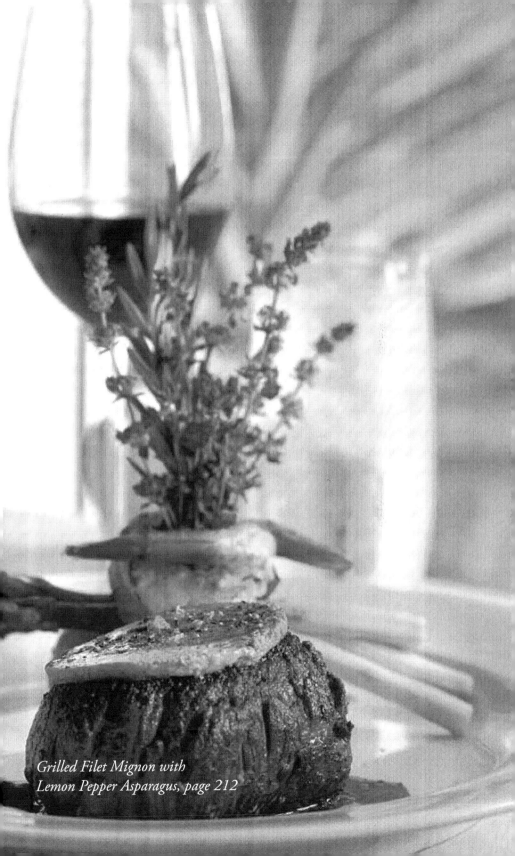

*Grilled Filet Mignon with
Lemon Pepper Asparagus, page 212*

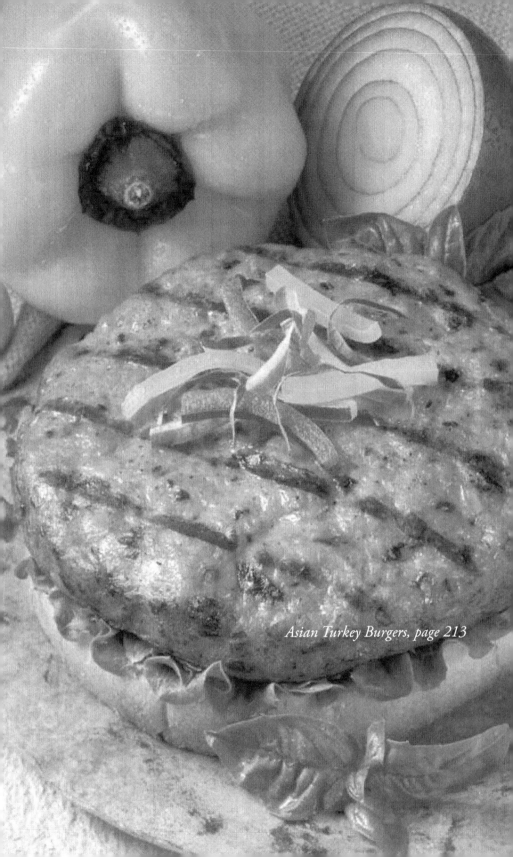

Asian Turkey Burgers, page 213

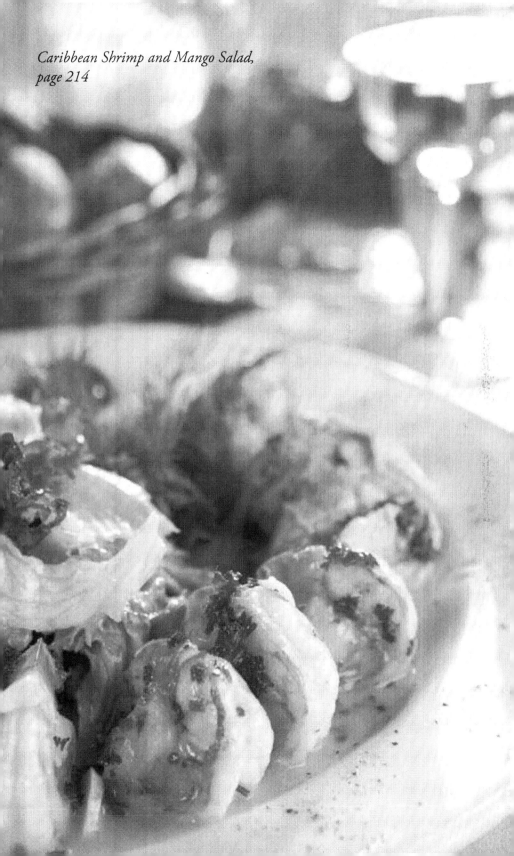
Caribbean Shrimp and Mango Salad,
page 214

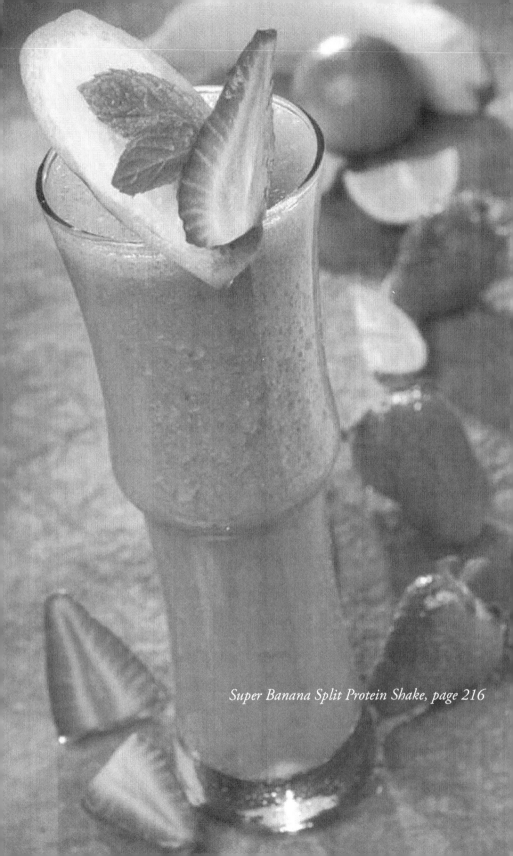

Super Banana Split Protein Shake, page 216

Ingredients

- 4 large red peppers cut in half
- Cold pressed extra virgin olive oil
- 2 Tbsp minced fresh basil
- 2 tsp balsamic vinegar
- Loaf of whole wheat bread, warmed to a light crisp in toaster oven
- Fresh minced Italian herbs: oregano, parsley, sage, rosemary, and thyme
- 1 clove garlic
- 24 piece of fresh shrimp, peeled and deveined

Directions

- Rub the peppers with olive oil and place on cookie sheet. Broil on high for about three to five minutes or until you see the skin bubble up brownish black. Take the peppers out and place inside a plastic bag. This is a top chef cooking trick, which will help you to take the skin off more easily. When the peppers are cool, rub off skin. In a bowl, place the meat of the pepper; add vinegar and seasoning. Serve on a colorful plate with the bread, or place peppers on top of the bread. In a heated skillet add cooking spray and slightly brown garlic. Add the shrimp, cooking three to four minutes until pink in color. Serve with peppers and bread.

BAKED BLACKENED SALMON STEAKS WITH MANGO AND BLACK BEAN SALSA

Salmon is one of my favorite fish, as it's loaded with Omega-3 fat, which is great for our hair, skin, and nails, and helps to fight off cancer. The fruit in the salsa adds a kick of sweetness and is loaded with vitamin C. The black beans add fiber and are rich in antioxidants.

Ingredients
- 1 large mango, pitted and diced into ½ inch pieces
- 1 kiwi, peeled and diced
- 1 can of black beans, rinsed and drained
- ¼ cup of cilantro, chopped
- 2 scallions, sliced tsp honey
- Dash of sea salt
- Dash of cayenne pepper
- 2 Tbsp salt-free blackening seasoning
- 1 lime, squeezed with juice set aside
- 4 salmon steaks, 4 ounces each

Directions
- Heat oven to 350 degrees. To make the salsa, in a mixing bowl, toss the first nine ingredients with half of the limejuice. Set the salsa aside. Place salmon steaks on a cooking tray. Drizzle the remaining juice over the fish. Sprinkle both sides with the blackening seasoning. Bake until cooked through, about fifteen to twenty minutes.

Mind, Body and Soul Diet Fit Tip: Always choose wild fish, never farmed. Farmed fish have higher levels of mercury and may even be toxic.

SUCCULENT AND EXOTIC ASIAN LETTUCE WRAPS

Bold flavors, crunchy vegetables, cool and crispy lettuce combined for delicious, hands-on meals! In addition, they're especially healthy. For lunch, add ½ cup cooked brown rice or a whole-grain roll for your complex carb. If you make this for dinner, eat without the carb.

Ingredients

- At least 16 Boston bib or butter lettuce leaves
- 1 pound lean ground turkey
- 1 large onion chopped
- 2 cloves fresh garlic minced
- 1 Tbsp low sodium soy sauce
- ¼ cup hoisin sauce
- 1 Tbsp rice wine vinegar
- Asian pepper chili sauce
- Dash of cayenne pepper
- 1 can water chestnuts, rinsed and drained
- 1 bunch green onions, finely chopped
- 2 tsp dark Asian sesame oil
- ¼ cup freshly minced parsley
- 1 Tbsp of chopped ginger

Directions

- Rinse lettuce leaves, pat dry. In a medium skillet over high heat, brown the ground turkey and then set aside. In the same pan, cook the onion in the same pan, stirring frequently. Add the garlic, soy sauce, hoisin sauce, ginger, vinegar, and chili pepper sauce to the onions and stir. Add water chestnuts, green onions, sesame oil, and cook for about two minutes until the onions begin to wilt. Stir in cooked ground turkey. Serve meat filling in a large bowl with the lettuce leaves on the side. Fill each lettuce leaf with the meat mixture and eat like a burrito. Enjoy the contrast of the crisp coolness of the lettuce leaf with the hot rich meat mixture inside.

FILET MIGNON WITH LEMON PEPPER ASPARAGUS

Sometimes your body needs a good steak. Lean red meat is high in protein, and has vitamins and minerals, such as iron and vitamin B12, that fish or poultry don't contain.

Ingredients
- 1 8 ounce lean filet mignon
- 1 tsp ground black pepper
- Horseradish, to serve on the side
- 8 to 10 large spears of asparagus
- Juice from one lemon
- Black pepper
- Olive oil

Directions
- Coat a nonstick pan with cooking spray. Heat to medium-high heat. Sprinkle pepper on both sides of steak. Place in pan, and sear on both sides. Cook to your liking. In a steamer, steam asparagus. Take out and drizzle with olive oil, squeeze the lemon on top, and then add a dash of freshly ground black pepper.

ASIAN TURKEY BURGERS

Here is a great recipe to liven up sometimes bland ground turkey. With garlic, parsley, ginger, and soy sauce, your burgers will be both delicious and packed with super food ingredients!

Ingredients
- 1 pound ground turkey
- 1 clove of garlic, finely minced
- ¼ cup minced onion
- 3 Tbsp chopped fresh parsley
- 2 Tbsp Worcestershire sauce
- 2 Tbsp minced green bell pepper
- 1 Tbsp low sodium soy sauce
- 1 Tbsp cold water
- 1 Tbsp grated fresh ginger
- ¼ tsp coarsely ground pepper
- 2 cloves of garlic crushed

Directions
- Combine all ingredients in a big bowl and mix together until they're well combined. Divide into three equal portions, and form into burgers about ¾ inch thick. Spray a skillet with nonstick cooking spray, and place over medium-high heat. Cook the burgers for about five minutes per side until done through. Top with freshly sliced tomatoes and cold crisp lettuce.

CARIBBEAN SHRIMP AND MANGO SALAD

Ingredients
- 1 lb medium shrimp peeled and deveined
- 2 cloves garlic, finely chopped
- 2 Tbsp Cold Pressed extra virgin olive oil
- 1 15 ounce can of black beans, rinsed and drained
- ¼ cup red onion, halved and then thinly sliced
- ½ cup of fresh lime and lemon juice, mixed together
- Dash of allspice
- 6 cups of mixed greens

Directions
- Cook shrimp with garlic in oil in skillet over medium low heat, not allowing the oil to smoke. Remove, and place in a large bowl. Add all other ingredients except the salad, tossing to coat. Then, just before serving, gently toss with the mixed greens.

Pre-bedtime Snack

- Small tin of tuna, rinsed, with a touch of fat free mayo and relish
- Two hard-boiled eggs with yokes removed, dashed with white pepper
- Small fat-free snack-size cottage cheese with strawberries and blueberries
- Chunks of cantaloupe wrapped in Prosciutto
- Four medium size precooked shrimp, dipped in cocktail sauce

Protein Shake Recipes

APPLE PIE À LA MODE PROTEIN SHAKE

Just like Mom used to make, but without the fat and calories!

Ingredients

- 8 ounces of cold water
- 1 scoop of BSN's Lean Dessert Protein Powder, Whipped Vanilla Flavor
- Dash of cinnamon
- Organic apple flavor extract
- 3 ice cubes
- 2 Tbsp Cool Whip Free

Directions

- Pour water into blender, then protein powder, dash of cinnamon, and apple flavor extract. Blend on high for one minute. Then add ice, blend on high for one minute more. Pour into glass, top with Cook Whip, and add another dash of cinnamon.

BEAUTIFUL BERRY BLAST PROTEIN SHAKE

Get a blast of antioxidant vitamin C, which is great for your immune system, plus gives you a super glow to your skin and helps to clear your complexion.

Ingredients

- 8 ounces of cold water
- 1 scoop of BSN's Lean Dessert Protein Powder, Whipped vanilla flavor

- 1 cup of blueberries, strawberries, raspberries, and blackberries

- 3 ice cubes

- 2 Tbsp of Cool Whip Free

- A few extra berries to put on top of whipped cream

- One sprig of mint

Directions

- Pour cold water into blender. Put protein powder and berries into blender, blend on high for one minute. Add ice cubes, and then blend on high for one minute. Pour into glass, top with Cool Whip and top with a few fresh berries and a spring of mint.

SUPER BANANA SPLIT PROTEIN SHAKE

Banana splits are my all-time favorite dessert! Here is a healthy version that gives you all the different flavors and tastes of a banana split, without the unnecessary calories, carbs, or sugar.

Ingredients

- 8 ounces of water

- One scoop of BSN's Lean Dessert Protein Powder, Banana Cream Flavor

- Half of one banana, or small banana

- Few chunks of fresh pineapple

- One maraschino cherry and a touch of its juice for that added "wow" factor, or fresh cherries, your choice

- 3 cubes of ice

Directions

- Blend on high and enjoy!

GERMAN CHOCOLATE CAKE PROTEIN SHAKE

There is nothing richer or dreamier than the combination of dark chocolate and the tropical scent of coconut. Another one of my favorite desserts, but this recipe will keep you lean while keeping you satisfied.

Ingredients
- 8 ounces of cold water
- 1 scoop of BSN's Lean Dessert Protein, Chocolate Coconut Candy Bar
- 1 Tbsp coconut oil
- 3 ice cubes
- Blend and enjoy!

Mind, Body and Soul Diet Fit Tip: Before you pour your shake into your glass, wet the rim with water and then dip it into coconut flakes. When you sip your shake, you will enjoy the scent and texture of the flakes on your rim for added pizzazz!

KEY LIME PIE PROTEIN SHAKE

I live in Miami, so when I get the chance to visit the Florida Keys, I stock up on fresh limes, which I use when I make this zesty and tangy shake.

Ingredients
- 8 ounces of cold water
- 1 scoop of BSN's Lean Dessert Protein shake, Whipped Vanilla Flavor
- Juice of one fresh lime
- ¼ cup of low-fat half and half
- 3 ice cubes

- 2 graham crackers, crushed up and placed in a dish

Directions
- Blend all ingredients on high, except the graham crackers. Wet rim of the glass with water, then dip into crushed graham crackers. Pour in protein shake mixture. Enjoy!

EXOTIC CHAI TEA PROTEIN SHAKE

This is a delicate blend of black tea, a touch of skim milk, ginger, and spices.

Ingredients
- 8 ounces of cold chai tea
- Dash of cinnamon
- Dash of ground ginger
- 1 scoop of BSN's Lean Dessert Protein Powder, Whipped Vanilla Flavor
- ¼ cup low fat half and half
- 3 ice cubes

Directions
- Blend on high speed and enjoy.

COOKIES AND CREAM PROTEIN SHAKE

An old-fashioned favorite reinvented with none of the guilt and a ton of health benefits.

Ingredients
- 8 ounces of cold water
- One scoop of BSN's Syntha 6, Cookies and Cream Flavored Protein Powder

- ¼ cup Cool Whip Lite
- 3 chocolate wafer cookies

Directions
- Add water to blender, add protein powder, and blend on medium speed until thoroughly mixed. Then add in Cool Whip, ice cubes and blend for about half a minute. Add cookie wafers and blend again for about fifteen seconds.
- Pour and enjoy!

ISLAND PINA COLADA PASSION

Send your taste buds into instant vacation mode with this tropical cooler.

Ingredient
- 8 ounces of water
- 1 scoop of BSN's Lean Dessert Protein Powder, Whipped Vanilla Flavor
- ¼ cup of fresh pineapple, cut into chunks
- 1 Tbsp of coconut oil

Directions
- Add water to blender, then add protein powder, ice cubes, pineapple chunks, and coconut oil. Whip on high until thoroughly blended. Pour and enjoy!

CHOCOLATE COVERED CHERRY PROTEIN SHAKE

What can be more irresistible, juicy, and luscious than a dark choco-late-covered cherry? Well, this protein shake, of course!

Ingredients
- 8 ounces of cold water
- 1 scoop of BSN's Lean Dessert Protein, Chocolate Fudge flavor
- 3 maraschino cherries
- 1 Tbsp of maraschino cherry juice (or you can opt for fresh-pitted cherries)
- 3 ice cubes

Directions
- Pour cold water into blender. Add protein powder, cherries, and ice. Blend on high.
- Pour and enjoy!

Mind, Body and Soul Diet Desserts

If you don't work in a dessert or two a week, you will feel deprived. So celebrate life's sweetness with my super healthy desserts that are just so good for you, that it would be sinful not to eat them!

GRILLED PEARS AND PEACHES WITH WARM WALNUT HONEY SAUCE

While pears and peaches are loaded with fiber, walnuts are loaded with omega-3 fats and blueberries are antioxidant powerhouses.

Ingredients
- Honey Dressing:
- 1 cup low fat vanilla yogurt
- 2 Tbsp honey
- 1 Tbsp fresh lemon juice
- 1 Tbsp coconut oil

Topping:
- ¾ cup chopped walnuts
- Unsweetened coconut flakes
- 1 pint of blueberries, washed
- ¼ cup chopped fresh mint
- 4 ripe pears
- 4 ripe peaches

Directions
- Preheat oven to 300 degrees. Whisk the yogurt, honey, coconut oil, and lemon juice in a small bowl. In another bowl, combine the blueberries and mint. Place in fridge until ready to use. Lightly brush pears and peaches with coconut oil and grill. Place grilled fruit in mixing bowl

with blueberries and mint. Evenly divide among four plates, drizzle with honey sauce and top with walnuts.

SICILIAN TIRAMISU

This is a super protein-packed dessert, loaded with antioxidants, vitamins, and minerals. It's rich, creamy, and naturally sweet! It has all the things a dessert should have, except all the extra calories, carbs, and sugar. The extra cocoa powder and delicious sweet strawberries add to the antioxidant punch that this dessert packs.

Ingredients
- 1 large container of fat free ricotta cheese
- Cocoa powder
- 5 tsp instant espresso powder or instant coffee powder
- 1 teaspoon Stevia
- 1 tsp vanilla extract
- Sugar-free/fat-free chocolate pudding
- Slivered roasted almonds
- 1 package of ladyfingers
- Fresh cut strawberries
- Fat-free whipped cream

Directions
- In a bowl mix the ricotta cheese, cocoa powder, almond, vanilla extract and Stevia.
- Set aside. In a small square dessert tray, layer the ingredients as follows: ladyfingers, ricotta mixture, sugar-free/fat-free chocolate pudding. Top with fat-free whipped cream and garnish with roasted slivered almonds and fresh strawberries.

BERRY RICH ANGEL FOOD CAKE

For when you are feeling like a little devil and need to please your sweet tooth! Full of antioxidant rich berries and omega-3 rich walnuts and protein-filled yogurt, this is a sinless dessert that your body will thank you for eating!

Ingredients
- Angel food cake
- Organic vanilla yogurt
- 2 cups each blueberries and strawberries
- Low-fat Cool Whip
- Walnuts

Directions
- Gently break up angel food cake with your fingers. Place one layer of angel food cake on bottom of a large glass dessert bowl. Layer with yogurt, berries, walnuts, and repeat. Top with low-fat Cool Whip, more berries, and walnuts.

Juice Recipes

Juicing is a quick, easy, and efficient way to give your body the vitamins and daily serving of fruits and vegetables that you need in one glass. And think about it—raw fruits and vegetables are living things! So if you want more energy, eat more of them. They are fresh, and haven't had their nutritional content diluted and diminished through cooking, processing, or being preserved. The more "alive" and "living" fresh fruits and vegetables you eat, the more alive you will feel and the more energy you will have! And when you incorporate such a blessing of nutrients into your food plan through juicing, you will enjoy heightened spiritual awareness, plus relaxation of the mind, body and soul. The combinations of fruit and vegetables are endless. Here are some of my favorite juice and veggie blends that will get and keep your body happy and humming. Cheers to your health!

BRAIN BOOSTER

Here is a juice to stimulate the other 90% of our brains that we don't use. This nutrient-rich, wide-spectrum juice will feed the brain into razor-sharp mode. The benefits of drinking this juice are better memory, acuity of mind, and a clearer head with no more morning brain fog. Put that bounce back into your step with this super juice!

- 1 pear
- 1 apple
- 1 orange
- 1 carrot stick
- 1 stalk celery
- 1 beet
- A small chunk of ginger
- Juice all ingredients and pour over ice. Drink immediately to get the best benefits.

PAIN-BE-GONE JUICE

To alleviate aches and pains, lessen irritation, and reduce inflammation, it's essential to detoxify the blood stream with super cleansing fruits and vegetables in a juice form for higher and quicker absorption. This juice is more than delicious, as it is also therapeutic and helps in the healing process. If you are waking up feeling stiff and suffer from arthritis, then this is a perfect blend of juices.

- 1 lemon
- 1 orange
- 1 pear
- 1 apple
- 1 pomegranate
- 1 large carrot stick
- A cup of fresh dark pitted cherries
- Juice all ingredients and pour over ice. Drink immediately to get the best benefits.

ATHLETE'S DELIGHT

If you want to start looking, feeling, and performing like an athlete, then you must fuel up like one! Enjoy this "lightening bolt" of energy in a glass that will help you to have more speed, agility, endurance, stamina, and quickness.

- 1 cup of watermelon
- 1 granny smith apple
- 1 lemon
- 1 cup of pineapple
- 2 stalks celery

- 1 cup of cantaloupe
- A small chunk of ginger
- A bunch of parsley
- Juice all ingredients and pour over ice. Drink immediately to get the best benefits.

ANTI-AGING JUICE RECIPE

Get a more youthful glow to your entire aura with this anti-aging super juice! And yes, antioxidants can help you turn back the clock!

- A handful of blueberries and strawberries
- A small bunch of parsley
- A healthy bunch of spinach and kale
- 1 kiwi
- 1 tomato
- 1 lemon
- 3 broccoli florets
- 1 apple
- 2 apricots
- 1 carrot
- 1 red pepper
- 2 beets
- Juice all ingredients and pour over ice. Drink immediately to get the best benefits.

FULL BODY CLEANSE AND BLOOD DETOXIFIER JUICE

Beets are the main focus of this juice because they're a powerful cleanser of the blood, kidneys, and liver. The garlic has doses of potassium, copper, iron, phosphorus, and iron, and will ward off any oncoming cold. The radish is a diuretic, cleanser, and disinfectant, which can help wash away the toxins accumulated in the kidneys.

- 1 garlic clove
- 4 beets
- 3 celery stalks
- 3 pineapple chunks
- A healthy amount of spinach
- 1 apple
- 1 piece of fresh ginger
- 1 tomato
- 4 radishes
- Juice all ingredients and pour over ice. Drink immediately to get the best benefits.

SEXY HAIR, SKIN, AND NAILS SIPPER

This beauty blend helps those of us who suffer from dull skin, dry hair, and easy-to-chip nails. This decadent sipper will give your outward appearance a healthy boost with juice to glow, radiate, and shine. Your skin will look brighter, your hair will be thicker and more lustrous, and your nails stronger. Being beautiful never tasted so good! Aloe is moisture-rich, and cucumber is high in silica, which is a mineral that fortifies connective tissue, thus increasing skin elasticity. Parsley promotes firming of the skin, and sweet potato is an excellent source of beta-carotene, which will give you a great complexion.

- 1 full aloe leaf

- 1 cucumber

- A handful of grapes

- 1 pomegranate

- A cup of blueberries and strawberries

- 1 sweet potato

- A few leaves of romaine lettuce

- A snip of parsley and parsnips

- Juice all ingredients and pour over ice. Drink immediately to get the best benefits.

The Power of Supplements

As a specialist in sports nutrition and supplementation, I clearly understand why it is absolutely essential to properly supplement. I know with conviction that nutritionally complementing your *Mind Body, and Soul Food Plan* with supplements, protein shakes, juices, vitamins, and minerals will help you enjoy optimal health.

In today's era of overly-processed food, many of the minerals and vitamins have been removed. A great way to add nutritional value where it has been taken away, is by supplementation. You will help to reverse your biological age, increase your stamina, energy, and endurance. Quite simply, supplements just make you look and feel healthier.

A word on protein supplements for lean muscle tone—it's essential to get adequate protein to help you build that sleek and sexy feminine muscle tone and also help rev up your metabolism. One way you can do that is through BSN supplements (to purchase, visit store.bsnonline.net). One of my favorite protein shakes is Lean Dessert Protein, and as you can see in the recipe section, I've got great protein shake recipes that you can whip up in a flash to have a whole, balanced meal in less than two minutes.

Vitamins and Minerals—
The Foundation

In order for your body to function optimally and remain healthy, you need a minimum amount of vitamins and minerals each day. Plain and simple, vitamins and minerals make people's bodies work properly. A balanced diet normally supplies sufficient vitamins. But really, who can honestly say they eat a balanced diet daily in today's hectic times?

Why is making sure you get enough vitamins and minerals in your diet so important in my Mind, Body and Soul Diet? Well, serious disorders can develop if your diet does not meet your body's needs. By the time a vitamin or mineral deficiency becomes apparent, the damage may already be done. Therefore, the key word here is "prevention." For example, people who do not have enough of the vitamins A, B1, and B2 are lethargic and emotionally or mentally disturbed. They have a poor appetite, and often suffer from dried lips, among other symptoms. The common causes of these vitamin deficiencies include bad eating habits, emotional stress, alcoholism, improper absorption of vitamins and minerals, the intake of medicines that interfere with the ingestion of vitamins, and lack of exposure to sunlight.

If you constantly feel tired and suffer from chronic health-related issues, you might be short of the vitamins that your body needs to function properly. Supplements address the lack of vitamins and minerals in the body.

Many have asked me if you still need to take vitamins even if you maintain a healthy diet. My answer is a resounding "yes!" Proper food consumption should be complemented with the right vitamins and minerals. Vitamins cover you in the event that your diet does not fully meet your daily requirements.

Vitamins fall into two categories: fat-soluble and water-soluble. The **fat-soluble** vitamins—A, D, E, and K—dissolve in fat and can be stored in your body. The **water-soluble** vitamins—C and the B-complex vitamins (such as vitamins B6, B12, niacin, riboflavin, and folate)—need to dissolve in water before your body can absorb them. Because of this, your body can't store these vitamins. Any vitamin C or B that your body doesn't use as it passes through your system is lost (mostly when you pee). So you need a fresh supply of these vitamins every day.

Whereas vitamins are organic substances (made by plants or animals), minerals are inorganic elements that come from the soil and water and are absorbed by plants or eaten by animals. Your body needs larger amounts of some minerals, such as calcium, to grow and stay healthy. Other minerals, like chromium, copper, iodine, iron, selenium, and zinc, are called trace minerals because you only need very small amounts of them each day.

There is an information overload on which vitamins and minerals need to be included in a healthy diet. It is often difficult to determine what is necessary and what is optional from the choices you have. I'm here to enlighten you and empower you—not confuse you. Therefore, I'm going to keep it simple and straight forward. I have compiled a short and sweet list of the ten most important vitamins your body needs.

1. Vitamin D deficiency can be quite dangerous. It leads to rickets in children, and osteoporosis and other diseases in adults. Vitamin D is very necessary for cancer prevention. In some places (Canada for instance), it is highly difficult to get enough Vitamin D from sunlight alone. Therefore, one needs to supplement the body with Vitamin D rich substances like vitamin D-fortified milk and milk substitutes, fatty fish such as salmon, and vitamin D-fortified yogurt.

2. Calcium, along with Vitamin D, is necessary for bone health. Low-fat or skim milk, low-fat dairy products, almonds, beans, sesame seeds, and broccoli are calcium-rich foods.

3. Women, especially at their pre-menopausal stage, need iron supplements. Fortified cereals, whole grains, dried fruits, nuts, and seeds are important sources of iron. Red meat is also rich in iron, but only three servings per week of it should be eaten. A combination of these iron supplements with ingredients high in Vitamin C will help your body absorb the iron properly.

4. Selenium is a lesser-known, but important, mineral. It supports the immune system, reduces inflammation and helps protect from cancer. Sunflower seeds, fish, shellfish, red meat, and one Brazil nut daily, will give you enough selenium. Selenium is also linked to reducing the risk of some cancers and is thought to possibly slow down the progression of HIV and AIDS. It also promotes excellent health by helping with normal liver function.

5. Vitamin C is an antioxidant vitamin that is believed to protect the brain from damage associated with Alzheimer's. It helps you to tackle stress better, and also protects you from common cold. A glass of orange juice, citrus fruits, bell peppers, kiwifruit, papaya, broccoli, dark leafy greens, and strawberries will provide you with Vitamin C.

6. Vitamin K plays an important role to strengthen the bones, avoid blood clotting and prevent hardening of arteries. Dark, leafy vegetables are good sources of Vitamin K.

7. Cancer-fighting B vitamin folate reduces the risk of Alzheimer's. It is good for pregnant women, as it reduces the risk of neural tube defects. Spinach provides you with folate. Other sources are beans, peanuts, broccoli, corn, lentils, and oranges.

8. The antioxidant Vitamin E fights free radicals and reduces risk of heart disease, stroke and Alzheimer's. Daily intake of nuts and seeds, such as almonds and sunflower seeds, will provide you with Vitamin E.

9. Magnesium is an important mineral that is often overlooked. In fact, up to 90 percent of Americans don't get the recommended daily allowance (RDA) of magnesium from their diet alone. Symptoms of magnesium deficiency can include leg cramps, migraines, fatigue, loss of appetite, depression, nausea and vomiting, or high blood pressure. The mineral Magnesium helps build strong bones and lowers the risk of diabetes by enhancing the action of insulin in your body. Beans, nuts, seeds, and green vegetables such as spinach are great sources of Magnesium.

10. Potassium helps to maintain blood pressure. It also helps reduce your risk of stroke. Beans, potatoes, sweet potatoes, bananas, dried fruits, winter squash, cantaloupe, kiwi, orange juice, prune juice, and avocados are good sources of Potassium.

The Smart Pills: Nutrients for Memory and Mental Well-Being

Your mind is your body's main "muscle." You must "feed" it positive thoughts and also, of course, feed it with memory-enhancing agents, like essential fatty acids, and also vitamins which help maintain mental sharpness. The herb Ginkgo Biloba is a memory- enhancing agent, and when digested can help increase mental performance. ALC, or acetyl-L-carnitine plays a special role in increasing the energy level of brain cells, which slows the progress of memory loss, and has also shown to help reduce symptoms of depression. Fatty fish, and also EFA's taken orally, have also been linked to mental well-being and mental acuity.

Ward Off the #1 Killer of Women with Supplements for the Heart

CoQ10 is a naturally-occurring compound found in the body, and a powerful antioxidant. It is a coenzyme, similar to a vitamin, and assists in various internal processes. Specifically, CoQ10 plays an essential role in the production of cellular energy. Without this energy, your cells cannot function. CoQ10 is found in high concentrations in tissues and organs that require a lot of energy. The heart requires huge amounts of energy to function, which is why CoQ10 is crucial in maintaining cardiovascular health. CoQ10 has been shown to help the function of the heart muscle and may also help those suffering from coronary heart disease, congestive heart failure, and also high blood pressure.

Keep Your Joints Juicy!

"You are only as old as your joints." — JNL

The more flexible you are, and the healthier your joints, the younger you feel, move around, and look. Chondroitin sulfate is in your cartilage. It brings fluid into the tissue to give our cartilage more elasticity and deters cartilage breakdown by protecting it from destructive enzymes. As a supplement, it is often taken along with Glucosamine to assist in maintaining joint health. The combined use is known to produce a synergistic effect. So make sure you feed your joints to stay feeling younger, and also aid in recovery from any joint injury.

Take the story of two completely different women into consideration, to help you realize just how important joint health is. Barb is 41, overweight with worn-out knees, and she has a hard time walking. Sue is 72, in shape with great flexibility, and her joints are in excellent condition. Who is really the older one? Who enjoys life more, with more physical freedom? You are only as old as your joints and as your body feels.

A Few of My Favorite Things...

"What's life without your favorite things?" — J N L

Being a highly sought after keynote speaker and author, as well as an international weight loss success story, I receive endless e-mails asking me what my favorite things are—the things I cannot live with and that I always use. Now I've got a complete list, just for you.

- *JNL's Favorite Brand of Organic Unrefined Coconut Oil:* Nutiva Extra Virgin Organic

- *JNL's Favorite Brand of Vitamins:* Solgar

- *JNL's Favorite Brand of ground flax blend:* Leonflax

- *JNL'S Favorite Brand of Cold-Press Extra Virgin Olive Oil:* Frantoia Olive Oil. This oil is made the old fashioned way with the Sicilian press.

- *JNL's Favorite brand of face care:* Yonka

- *JNL's Favorite Brands of skin firming, cellulite fighting, and stretch mark repair lotions:* Clarins

- *JNL's Favorite brand for yogurt drink:* DanActive Low Carb by Dannon

- *JNL's Favorite brand light yogurt:* Stoneyfield's Organic

- *JNL's Favorite brands of extra dark chocolate:* Lindt 85% Cocoa Extra Fine Dark Chocolate is great because you can find it at your local convenience store or grocery. There are also many great antioxidant rich dark chocolates on the market, which will help keep you satisfied and also speed up the process of your weight loss. Just look for over 70% cocoa.

- *JNL's Favorite Powder Vitamin C Mix for Water:* Emergen-C

- *JNL's Favorite Lo-Carb Whole Wheat Tortillas:* Tam-x-kos

- *JNL's Favorite Bran Muffin Mix:* Duncan Hines All-Bran Muffin Mix. It's made with Kellog's All-Bran, and have fun with adding your favorite nuts or dried fruit to the mix. Visit www.duncanhines.com

- *JNL's Favorite Light Cheese:* Babybel Light Cheese—all of the flavors! www.laughingcow.com

- *JNL's Favorite Line of Fitness Supplements:* Lean Dessert Protein, Syntha 6, and Atro-Phex by BSN. Being a modern-day, multitasking businesswoman and mother, I don't have a lot of time to waste. BSN's entire line of high quality supplements allows me to "lean out" quicker, blast fat faster, and maintain my weight loss in an easier and more manageable manner. As you can see in my recipe section, I rely on these super rich and thick protein shakes. BSN's proteins and nutrients save me time and energy, and enable me to maintain my weight loss goals. Visit www. BSNOnline.net

- *JNL's Favorite Exercise DVDs:* When I'm long on needing a workout and short on time, I love to pop in an exercise DVD and press play. My favorites are available at www. AbCirclePro.com and also ShopJNL.com.

- *JNL's Favorite Exercise Equipment:* Ab Circle Pro is a fantastic tool that has helped me burn fat and calories and chisel out my core without having to get on the floor and do another sit-up. It allows me to get in a quick three to five-minute workout to keep my six-pack abs in check and stay camera ready. The Ab Circle Pro is available at www. AbCirclePro.com.

- *JNL's Favorite Hair Care:* Creo Hair Care is absolutely the best, and it's the exclusive line that I trust my tresses with. It's sulfate free, all natural, paraben free, DEA and TEA free, vegan, and it preserves my hair protein. Check out their amazing product line and why it's so special at GetCreoNow.com.

- *JNL's Favorite Fitness Programs:* My FitnessModelProgram. com is an amazing way to lose weight and gain strength at home or at the gym with my tried and true top fitness model secrets, workouts, and recipes. I have taken all of the guesswork out and given you the exact guide you need to follow to get the results you want. You will look and feel like a super strong, sexy, bold, athletic super fitness model, as your body will be a fierce force to be reckoned with. If you want to get the body that looks as if it jumped off the cover of a top fitness magazine, then check out FitnessModelProgram.com.

If you need to bring sexy back, get your groove on, or you've figured out that your mojo isn't mojo'ing anymore, then visit TheSexyBodyDiet.com. I created this program for all the women who have been silently suffering in their own sensuality, and who don't remember the last time they felt attractive, beautiful, desired, and sexy. This is a program that all women must read.

CONCLUSION

Rome Wasn't Built in a Day

"Give yourself the gift of time."

—JENNIFER NICOLE LEE

I love the old adage that Rome wasn't built in a day, because it really sums up why the Mind, Body and Soul Diet works. I'm sure you've been where I was. You've done it quick, you've done it through the band-aid approach, only to find yourself back where you started.

This time, it's going to be different. This time, you're working with tried and true, foolproof, universal truths that will help you work smarter not harder, get maximum results, and enjoy the process—in all areas of your life. You're going to allow yourself the gift of time to have this new, improved quality lifestyle and body. You've planted the seeds of prosperous principles, and with time they will grow, flourish, and create priceless fruit, which are all the great blessings to come in your life.

I want to give you one final formula. There are three Fs that equal an A in working out and also in life: focus, form, and fun!

Focus on your immediate task at hand, which is helping yourself. Then let that trickle to others in your life when they are ready for it. Don't cheat yourself by trying to take a shortcut. Go from point A to point B utilizing all of the success principles I've given you.

Make sure you have proper form when you're doing your workouts, and even when you're using your success principles.

And lastly, have fun! It must be fun to work out, or you won't stick with it. Remember that empowering question I posed, "How can I work out and enjoy it?" Your mind will give you the answer!

It's important to protect your new, empowered, and enlightened lifestyle from the "weeds." When you start seeing results materialize in your life, it's common practice to get scared. It's called "approach/avoidance," remember? I'm urging you; do not press the rewind button. You cannot move forward by continuously looking in your rearview mirror. Allow the journey to take you to the destination to which you have desired to go for so long.

Maybe you have to hit your head against the wall just one more time; maybe you haven't hit the threshold of pain like my other weight loss clients have, like I did, that made us finally do it the right way. I can't tell you the exact amount of time it will take for you to start seeing results. But, I can guarantee you this: if you're persistent in implementing the Mind, Body and Soul Diet principles in your life that I've outlined in the past chapters, you will get results—and the results will be not temporary. There will be a lifelong domino effect.

You will no longer function out of a mindset of fear; you will now be functioning out of a mindset of the F-word, faith, that priceless mindset that any and all things are possible through your Higher Power, with the right tools and guidelines. You will no longer be silently suffering and asking yourself, "Am I doing this for all the wrong reasons?" Now, you'll lose weight for the right reasons: to help yourself and others around you. So don't get caught up in how long it takes to get the results you want.

Remember my story? I started my own weight loss journey and transformational program and almost threw in the towel because I didn't see results fast enough. It's human nature. Even I said, "The scale hasn't budged in two and a half months. I'm not dropping in dress sizes. I don't feel fit. I'm just doing this for vanity's sake. I'm kind of lost here." But my Higher Power answered me and told me to continue.

So I'm urging you to never give up, and never give in. Give yourself the gift of time so that your new, healthy lifestyle has a chance to materialize. Ultimately, you will see the results you want, but it is so much more important to enjoy the journey. You didn't start walking overnight, you didn't start talking overnight; it's the same thing with your new lifestyle and your new principles. Practice, persist, and always keep your eye on the prize.

Coaching Programs

"The correct information is priceless."
—JENNIFER NICOLE LEE

During one of my latest key media appearances, the interviewer looked me in the eye and asked, "How important is hiring a life coach, and why is coaching important?"

I was boggled by this question. The interviewer was questioning whether life coaching actually produces results. My answer is this: life coaching is absolutely essential. In this dog-eat-dog world, where it's pretty much survival of the fittest, you have to know what to do to get ahead of the pack, break away from all the wannabes, and set yourself up as a doer. Even the most successful athletes, the top strategic minds of tech empires, and the most amazing mixed martial artists in the UFC rely upon life coaches to give them that cutting, winning edge.

I can tell you that I would probably be light years ahead of where I am right now if I had truly understood the importance of life coaches ten years ago. If I had embraced my ability to hire a coach and not tried to do it the hard way, I would not have wasted so much time, money, and energy before I figured it out.

The problem is that a lot of people are close-minded; they're afraid to try to new techniques that have actually been proven to work, and they shun the metaphysical approach that the top coaches use. My point is this; to get results, you have to be highly coachable. You've got to listen to the experts.

So many people have the right intentions, but are using belief systems that were passed down to them. I hate to say it, but your parents paradigms are not what's happening in today's multitasking, information-in-an-instant age. In this new era, you need to be equipped with the latest, most innovative way to produce results. One of my favorite books, *Who Moved My Cheese?*, puts it this way: you must adapt and be flexible because there is only one constant in life, and that's change. You must be able to work with change and focus on how to streamline your results. But who's going to give you those answers? Life coaches; people who have done it before.

Once you fully understand how important life coaching is, that is the time for you to implement what you know. I pride myself in providing a top-of-the-line coaching program, The Mind, Body and Soul Program, to help you lose weight and gain a new identity as a healthy, super-fit athlete; to help you de-clutter yourself mentally; to help you get rid of self-sabotaging behaviors; and help you create a business out of your own true passions. If you don't know what your passions are anymore, I will help you reawaken them.

You can access the complete coaching services I provide at JenniferNicoleLee.com. I have a complete menu of different coaching programs that is designed to help you find the one that's right for you.

- If you want to increase your productivity and efficiency, you can do a one-on-one coaching consultation with me at ClubJNL.com.

- If you want to look like a fitness model, you can go to FitnessModelProgram.com.

- If you want to look like you just walked out of a bikini catalog, not as rock hard as a fitness model, you can go to BikiniModelProgram.com.

- If you want to reawaken your inner goddess, reconnect with your sensual side, and get your "sexy" back, you can do that with my innovative, unique, sensually reawakening program entitled TheSexyBodyDiet.com.

- If you're looking for a complete four-week, twenty-eight-day guide to take you by the hand and tell you what to eat, how to train, and even equip you with motivational quotes, positive affirmations, and powerful visualization exercises, visit GetFitNowwithJNL.com.

- If you're looking to really blast fat and rev your metabolism, you can visit JNLCracktheCode.com.

- If you have all the right intentions and are still not seeing results, I have an amazing eBook, *101 Things Not to Do*, available at 101ThingsNottoDo.com. The concept behind the book is that the things you're doing now, thinking they're healthy for you, are actually sabotaging your efforts.

- And if you want to improve the quality of your lifestyle in all areas, you can visit MindBodyandSoulProgram.com.

So, as you can see, I have a program designed especially for you and your desired outcome.

The Mind, Body and Soul Program

"Get where you belong." — J N L

Have you ever wondered why some people are able to achieve success in their lives, even if they experienced humble or harsh conditions growing up? They had no support system; they had no real role models or anyone to look up to; they had no financial support to help them achieve. Well, the answer is to be found in success principles, and you've been exposed to a lot of them in *The Mind, Body & Soul Diet.*

The accompanying online guide to this book, The Mind, Body and Soul Program, will provide you with more of the answers you're looking for. It's designed especially for people who believe they deserve more, and are hungry for more in all areas of their lives—which is you!

We live in the information age. Information is priceless, and information can give you results. If you want to use the same success principles that have helped me, as well as thousands of other women around the world, log onto MindBodyandSoulProgram.com. It's an online fitness, life, and business coaching program that's a click away. The great thing about it is that you have me "coming to you" in five one-hour-long audio seminars designed to equip you with empowering and enlightening tips, tools, and techniques to help you get where you belong.

How does The Mind, Body and Soul Program differ from *The Mind, Body & Soul Diet?* In addition to four seminars on the mind and emotional state, the body, and the soul, I add a fifth audio seminar to help you create financial prosperity in these dry economic times. It's as simple as logging onto the Internet and entering your contact information. You'll be equipped with my personal words to help you make your mind your best friend and not your worst enemy, by ending all negative self-talk and poor self-image. You'll learn how to stop emotional eating forever. You'll learn how to increase your productivity, efficiency, and effectiveness in all areas of your life. And finally, you'll lose weight and gain the new healthier lifestyle that you want.

The opportunities and advantages that past Mind, Body and Soul Program members have enjoyed are now available to you, to help you take action in your life. Stop working hard for your money and start creating money. Stop living in scarcity and start living in unlimited abundance. Do what you want to, and do it now. Gain clarity. Learn how to set goals that will really work. Gain the persistence you need, and never give up on your dreams of transforming yourself for success.

MY MIND, BODY & SOUL
DIET JOURNAL

Here is your private area for you to jot down your inner thoughts and feelings, hopes & dreams! Remember, "Thoughts become things," so dare to dream big!

_____

_____

_____

_____

_____

_____

_____

_____

_____

_____

_____

_____

_____

_____

_____

_____

_____

_____

_____

_____

_____

_____

_____

_____

MY MIND, BODY & SOUL
DIET BEFORE PHOTO

Take your "before" photo and tape or glue it here. Look at this photo daily, and remind yourself that this is the old you, and you are now working faithfully to create the new & improved, healthy, healed & happy you!

MY MIND, BODY & SOUL
DIET AFTER PHOTO

Place your "after" photo here. Have fun browsing through magazines and/ or the internet and find your favorite body and fitness level you would love to have one day. Look at this photo daily, and tell yourself that you can do it, and you will!

MY MIND, BODY &
SOUL DIET NOTES

Here is a special and sacred place for you to jot down notes, write down your goals, and to draft out your future success plans, with no one to judge you or critique you! Use this area to highlight areas of the book which especially struck you. Visit back here daily to reinforce what you have learned.

_____

_____

_____

_____

_____

_____

_____

_____

_____

_____

_____

_____

_____

_____

_____

_____

_____

_____

_____

_____

_____

_____

_____

_____

_____

_____

_____

Jennifer Nicole Lee

Jennifer Nicole Lee is one of the world's most accomplished entrepreneurial CEO's. Thanks to her successful internationally broadcast infomercial and media appearances, she is a household name in over 90 different countries, with her fitness messages translated in over 20 different languages. She is an international fitness celebrity, bestselling author, highly sought-after motivational keynote speaker, certified life coach, Team BSN athlete, and a Specialist in Sports Nutrition and Supplementation, with a focus on anti-aging. Her international and inspirational weight loss success story has motivated millions to take action in their own lives. Her cutting edge yet timeless lifestyle fitness expertise has been featured on *The Oprah Winfrey Show, The Big Idea with Donny Duetsch*, E! Entertainment, *Inside Edition, Fox & Friends, CBS Early Morning Show*, and WE Entertainment's *Secret Lives of Women*. She has been featured in countless magazines and editorials and is regarded as one of the world's top fitness celebrities, thanks to her remarkable image of health, vibrancy, youth, and glamour. JNL is a regular featured fitness expert and celebrity on the HSN Chanel, sharing her favorite wellness, fitness, and lifestyle products. She is the CEO of JNL, Inc., a company she founded with the mission statement: "I will share and shine my light to help others realize and then achieve their lifestyle goals, as I believe that everyone deserves to increase the quality of their lives." Jennifer lives in Miami with her husband, Edward, and sons Jaden Byron and Dylan Edward.

You can visit Jennifer Nicole Lee at her website:
www.**JenniferNicoleLee**.com

Made in the USA
Lexington, KY
15 April 2013